MW00632374

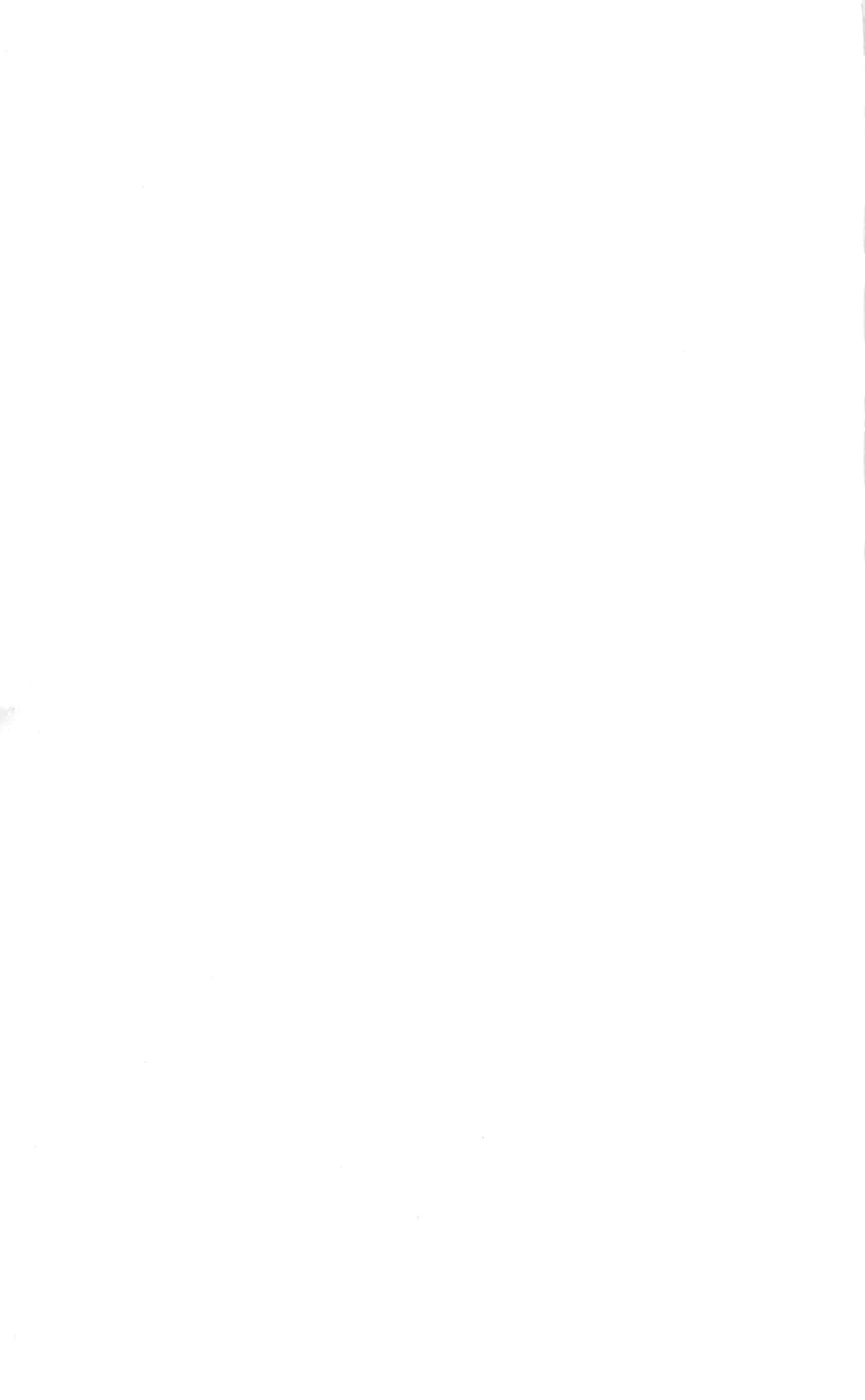

A MANUAL OF MILITARY SURGERY,

FOR THE USE OF

SURGEONS IN THE CONFEDERATE ARMY;

WITH AN APPENDIX OF THE

Rules and Regulations of the Medical Department

OF THE

CONFEDERATE ARMY.

BY

J. JULIAN CHISOLM, M. D.,

PROFESSOR OF SURGERY IN THE MEDICAL COLLEGE OF THE STATE OF SOUTH CAROLINA, ETC.

CHARLESTON:

EVANS & COGSWELL, No. 3 BROAD STREET.

1861.

PREFACE.

In putting forth this Manual of Military Surgery for the use of surgeons in the Confederate service, I have been led by the desire to mitigate, if possible, the horrors of war as seen in its most frightful phase in military hospitals. As our entire army is made up of volunteers from every walk of life, so we find the surgical staff of the army composed of physicians without surgical experience. Most of those who now compose the surgical staff were general practitioners, whose country circuit gave them but little surgery, and very seldom presented a gunshot wound. Moreover, as our country had been enjoying an uninterrupted state of peace, the collecting of large bodies of men, and retaining them in health, or the hygiene of armies had been a study without an object, and therefore without interest. When the war suddenly broke upon us, followed immediately by the blockading of our ports, all communication was cut off with Europe, which was the expected source of our surgical information. As there had been no previous demand for works on military surgery, there were none to be had in the stores, and our physicians were compelled to follow the army to battle without instruction. No work on military surgery could be purchased in the Confederate States. As military surgery, which is one of expediency, differs so much from civil practice, the want of proper information has already made itself seriously felt. In times of war, where invasion threatens, every citizen is expected to do his duty to his state. I saw no better means of showing my willingness to enlist in the cause than by preparing a manual of instruction for the use of the army, which might be the means of saving the lives and preventing the mutilation of many friends and countrymen. The present volume contains the fruit of European experience, as dearly purchased in recent campaigning. Besides embodying the experience of the masters in military surgery as to the treatment of wounds, I have incorporated chapters upon the food, clothing and hygiene of troops; with directions how the health of an army is to be preserved, and how an effective strength is to be sustained; also, the duties of military surgeons, both in the camp and in the field. In an appendix will be found the regulations and forms for the use of the Medical Department of the Confederate army. In preparing this volume, I have not hesitated to add to my own experience in the treatment of surgical injuries, any useful information which I could obtain from the most recent German, French and English works, on military surgery; and in many instances, where the language used by them expressed to the point the subject under discussion, I have not hesitated to transfer entire sentences directly to these pages. I make this acknowledgment, *en masse*, of the very liberal use of the following works, as quotation marks were sometimes overlooked:

Maximen der Kriegsheilkunst, von L. Stromeyer, Hanover, 1855; supplement der Maximen der Kriegsheilkunst, von L. Stromeyer, Hanover, 1860; Loeffler Behandlung der Schusswunde, Berlin, 1859; Histoire Médico-Chirurgicale de la Guerre de Crimée, par le docteur Adolphe Armand, Paris, 1858; La Guerre de Crimée, par L. Baudens, Paris, 1858; Des Plaies d'Armes a feu; Communications—Faites a l'Académie Nationale de Médecine, Paris, 1849; Notes of the Wounded, from the

Mutiny in India, by George Williamson, London, 1859; Coles' Military Surgery, with Experience of Field Practice in India, London, 1852; Gunshot Wounds of the Chest, by Patrick Fraser, M. D., London, 1859; Guthrie's Commentaries on Military Surgery, London, 1855; McLeod's Notes on the Surgery of the Crimean War, London, 1858; Hennen's Principles of Military Surgery; Larrey's Military Surgery; Ballingall's Outlines of Military Surgery; Gross' System of Surgery; Erichsen's Science and Art of Surgery; Jackson on the Formation, Discipline, and Economy of Armies.

INDEX.

CHAPTER I.

The Physical and Medical Topography of the Frontier States—Maryland, Virginia, Kentucky, Tennessee, Illinois and Missouri—their Geology, Climate, and Diseases; at what seasons prevalent, and how treated by the local physicians.

The war which is now being carried on between the United States and Confederate States has located itself, as it were by mutual consent, upon the frontier, which threatens to be the scene of most of the battles between the contending armies. As the middle region of what was formerly called the United States will witness the brunt of these contests, a brief description of the country, with a history of the diseases most prevalent at different seasons of the year, cannot but interest those who will have the sanitary condition of our troops under care; as it may assist army surgeons in adopting a system of hygiene and prophylactics which will be useful in keeping off diseases.

MARYLAND, the first of these border States upon the Atlantic coast, is naturally divided into two distinct physical regions: the one, an elevated region, traversed by various ridges of the Alleghanies, the other, a flat country, scarcely rising above the level of the sea, which in turn is cleft unequally by the Chesapeake bay. The lowlands on either side of the bay are more or less sandy, and are freely indented by estuaries and checkered by water courses. That portion of the State bordering on the Chesapeake is formed of lowlands and meadows. On the margin of these are salt marshes of considerable extent. Many of these are inundated by high tides, especially after the prevalence of south winds, which force the waters of the Chesapeake and its branches toward its sources. As the tides recede, many pools are left, which in hot weather form stagnant foci of infection. The lowlands are covered with a rank growth, the decomposition of which during the summer and autumn months charges the atmosphere with offensive and deleterious effluvia. Along these water courses and in the neighborhood of such lowlands, malaria abounds, and intermittent and remittent fevers are endemic.

The climate, as in all Southern latitudes, is very variable upon the coast, and the excessive moisture in an exhilarating atmosphere, when connected with the heats of summer, predispose to affections of the mucous membranes. The warm weather induces engorgements of the portal and hepatic circulation, with consequent derangement and interruption of the biliary secretion, with congestion and irritability of the intestinal mucous membrane. The sudden changes of temperature, making a rise or fall of several degrees of the thermometer, often in a few minutes, when taken in connection with suppression of perspiration, will explain the frequency of gastric disturbances, with diarrhœa and dysentery. These form the common diseases of the country during the summer months, and impress, to a greater or less extent, all morbid conditions.

As the land recedes at some distance from the bay, it becomes uneven. It gradually rolls into upheaved hills, the highest of which are not over one hundred feet in height. As the western portions of the State are approached, the land becomes very hilly and rough. The high ridges, which attain an elevation of 2,000 feet above the level of the sea, intercept valleys remarkable for the exuberant richness of the soil, which lies upon a substratum of limestone. This is the mining portion of the State, which yields coal in great abundance, and also iron. The water of this region is very free from impurities, whether obtained from the numerous streams, wells, or springs. Mineral waters are found in several localities, to many of which invalids resort with benefit. During the summer months, the highlands of the State are very healthy; and, except upon the low margins of the water courses, where the mild forms of malarial fevers are met with, no diseases can be called local. During the winter months, catarrhal affections and pneumonia are the diseases of the low countries, whilst typhoid fever often rages as an epidemic in the highest regions of the State.

Malarial fevers of this region commence their incursions about the middle of July, and continue three or four months. They take on either remittent or intermittent forms, and are of every grade of intensity, from the fevers of a day to those fatal after three or four paroxysms. Intermission or remission is their never-failing characteristic, by which they can always be recognized, and their lurking influence over other diseases detected. In later years these fevers have assumed a more manageable type, and yield readily to quinine when given early and in sufficient quantity.

Dysentery occurs annually in both the high and low portions of the country, and in some seasons assumes the epidemic character. When this disease appears during the autumn months, its association with malarious influences can be discerned, and the treatment, which is tedious, must be modified more or less on account of this combination. When the fever which accompanies this intestinal disease shows a periodic tendency more or less marked, the curative power of quinine in its treatment is proved to be of decided utility.

Catarrhal fevers often prevail extensively over large districts of country, owing, perhaps, to the presence of some subtle poison in the air which has eluded scientific inquiry. When prevalent, it brings under its influence almost every person in those districts where it makes its appearance. The course of the disease is to recovery after tormenting its victims from one to six weeks, and then leaving them much enfeebled. The mild expectorant plan of treatment is the course generally pursued by the local physicians, except where periodicity shows itself, when a few doses of the potent medicine, quinine, may, as if by magic, restore the patient to health.

VIRGINIA similates, closely, Maryland as to its topography. The coast line, running inward for one hundred to one hundred and twenty miles, is low and sandy, similarly indented with estuaries, into which the numerous rivers of the State empty. The lagoons are lined by low, marshy swamps, in which, during the summer months, malaria is generated. As we leave this belt, advancing westward, the country is found undulating, with rolling lands. The soil is somewhat sandy, but on the margins of the rivers are extensive alluvions of great fertility, producing fine crops of grain and tobacco, and supporting a healthy, sturdy population. The climate is salubrious, although variable. Traversing the centre of the State from north-east to south-west is the Blue Ridge and Alleghany chain of high mountains, rich in mineral productions, and enclosing fertile valleys, which will vie with any lands on the continent in productiveness. These valleys are filled with medicinal springs of great virtue. Many are of world-wide reputation, and are annually resorted to by thousands for health and pleasure. Among them are found lime, soda, sulphur, magnesia, alum, and chalybeate waters; also, hot, warm and cold springs. As the beautiful scenery, the bracing air, and excellent accommodations have their sanitary influence, especially when assisted by the medicinal waters which abound everywhere through these mountain ranges, the sick and halt from the most distant portions of the country are assembled here during the summer months. Nor are they often disappointed in the cures which they seek. Change of life and scene is a most potent remedy for good to those whose multifarious duties at home are constantly at war with all the laws of health.

WESTERN VIRGINIA, like the eastern portion of the State of KENTUCKY, with which it joins, is a broken country, abounding in the finest limestone water. The soil is fertile, based upon a substratum of blue limestone, which forms the basis of this entire region. In some portions, the soil is a rich black loam, and very productive ; in other portions, there is a red, yellowish or whitish clay, not so well adapted for grain crops. When a substratum of clay is covered with a layer of vegetable mould, it constitutes a soil of unrivalled fertility, in which the blue grass (*poa pratensis*) grows in the greatest perfection. A strong similarity exists between the diseases of this section, including Kentucky and those of the eastern portion of the State. Malarial fevers are of a mild type, and are found very amenable to treatment. It is chiefly where from freshets the rivers overflow their banks, leaving deposits to be acted upon by the hot sun of summer, that malaria is generated. In many low portions of Tennessee and Kentucky, in the neighborhood of the low banks of the rivers, the sources of malaria are found producing virulent cases of fever.

The western portions of TENNESSEE and KENTUCKY, with the southern part of ILLINOIS, are low river bottoms of rich soil, covered with rank vegetation. This portion of Illinois, skirting the Mississippi river for sixty miles in length and seven in width, is known as "the great American bottom." The immediate banks of the river, from one-half to one mile in depth, are bordered by a heavy forest, behind which margin is a rich prairie country, covered with luxuriant crops of grass. This prairie is dotted with numerous lakes, and as the evaporation of the water during the latter part of summer exposes the surface of the subjacent soil, a fruitful source of disease is engendered. The influence of this poisoned atmosphere is so sensibly felt on the opposite side of the river, which is here one mile wide, that at Jefferson barracks—a beautifully located station in a rolling, thoroughly drained country, gradually rising into hills at an elevation of two hundred feet, and one mile distance from the river bank—nearly all the garrison are affected by malarial fevers during the fall months. The medical statistics of the United States army give, as the annual average sickness for twenty-one years at this post, eight hundred and eighty-four cases of malarial fevers per thousand men. These statistics are gathered from a mean strength of nine thousand six hundred and eighty-one men.

At this station, intestinal diseases are very prevalent during warm weather. The proportion of these, exclusive of Cholera Asiatica, amounting to eight hundred and nine per thousand. Asiatic Cholera has raged at this post as an epidemic for several consecutive summers, having appeared in 1849, '50, '51, '52, '54 and '55.

Among the common diseases of this entire range of country, extending through all the middle States from the seaboard to the Mississippi, can now be classed Erysipelas. For the past ten or twelve years it has been found very prevalent, especially during the winter months, when the disease appears more severe. This, with Typhoid Fever, which, as a disease of the winter season, is also common to this entire belt of country, is of comparatively recent introduction. The former inflammatory character of diseases has given place to lower types, with increased irritability of the system, with its accompanying intolerance of antiphlogistic treatment and urgent demands for protection and stimulation.

The diseases which an army must encounter during the summer months, when encamped on the soil of Maryland, Virginia, Kentucky or Missouri, will depend altogether upon its location, whether on the low or high lands. If in the low country, in the vicinity of water courses, malarial fevers may be the most numerous, their frequency depending upon the degree of exposure. These are found to be amenable to treatment, and quinine is the great specific for this common disease. The majority of uncomplicated cases will, according to the experience of local physicians, yield to a single dose of ten to fifteen grains, given ten hours before the expected paroxysm. To those who are especially exposed in scouting parties or in the swamps, the prophylactic influence of quinine should be extensively relied upon, and cannot be too strongly urged. Five grains, taken daily, has proved sufficient protection on the river swamps of South Carolina, where malaria in its most concentrated and virulent forms infests the atmosphere.

When we leave the coast line and reach the hilly country, we come to a genial climate and salubrious country, where general health can be preserved. No malarial influences are here felt except upon the alluvial banks of the rivers, where it is sometimes met with in a mild form during the autumn months. Here Diarrhœa and Dysentery will be the prevailing affections, with gastric disturbances, and perhaps cholera morbus. These intestinal diseases often rage epidemically over extensive tracts, as found in Reports to the American Medical Association. All of the Middle States are common ground for these general diseases, which commence in June and continue until October, increasing in severity with the advance of hot weather. Even among the mountain ranges, with the most salubrious climate, diarrhœa shows itself the prevailing disease. From the medical reports of Carlisle barracks and Alleghany arsenal, extending over a series of years, and which have been compiled by order of surgeon-general Lawson, we find the proportion of Diarrhœa in the garrison to number, annually, five hundred and sixty-two per thousand, and Intestinal affections, exclusive of Asiatic Cholera, to be one thousand and seven cases per thousand men.

Exposure to atmospheric vicissitudes, eating crude and indigestible articles of food, unripe fruits and vegetables, intemperance in eating and drinking, irregularity in eating, improper clothing, with sudden check of perspiration, are the common productive causes of intestinal disturbances.

These diseases show no peculiarity; they are rarely purely inflammatory, and seldom demand the strictly antiphlogistic plan of treatment. Opium forms the basis of treatment for most bowel complaints, in combination with a little calomel to excite secretions from the liver, and also ipecac in small doses to restore cutaneous action, and perhaps camphor, for its general stimulating effect. By the judicious use of these remedies, intestinal fluxes are readily controlled.

When, from the enervating effects of long-continued heat, with its sedative influence upon the skin, these diseases assume a chronic form, a furlough for two or three weeks, with change of air, when assisted with mild astringent tonics, will be found the most successful treatment. The modern treatment of Dysentery by salines and opiates has called for many advocates, who use largely salts and laudanum as a prescription for it; the object being to relieve the engorgement of the vessels with the saline laxative, whilst the opiate allays irritability and checks tormina and tenesmus. Judging from an analysis of the reports handed in from the various Middle States to the American Medical Association, there is no very great difference in the success of these two modes of treatment. External stimulation by dry heat;

cataplasms of mustard or cayenne pepper; frictions, in connection with internal stimulation by administering the æthers, Hofmann's anodyne, spirits of camphor, essence of peppermint, ginger or tincture of capsicum, become very necessary when exhaustion of the nervous powers and collapse, with cold extremities, make their appearance.

In western Tennessee and Kentucky during the summer months malarial fevers are found, assuming a bilious remittent or intermittent type. They are amenable to the judicious administration of the preparations of bark, of which quinine and cinchona are the most active.

During the winter months, the high region of these Middle States becomes the most unhealthy. Catarrhal affections prevail upon the coast, now and then, taking on pneumonic symptoms; but with these, when not neglected in the commencement, there is no fatal tendency. In the mountain lands, Typhoid Fever may be expected, sometimes raging extensively and fatally. It is often the leading disease of the season. It generally runs a uniform course, ending when skilfully treated, in convalescence in from fourteen to twenty-one days. In its treatment, the intractable and depressing nature of the disease must be kept continually in view; the aim of the physician being rather to brace up the system against the exhausting effects of the disease and allow it to run its course. All depressing agents, as the mercurial preparations, etc., are thought prejudicial when given for their peculiar effect. Quinine has not proved itself so useful in controlling the febrile paroxysms, as might have been supposed, unless the fever shows a marked remission. Opium in guarded doses is found invaluable in controlling the looseness of the bowels, in quieting delirium and inducing sleep. The bowels, when a tendency to constipation exists, are kept soluble by the mild cathartics, as rhubarb, magnesia or castor oil, with a little turpentine; and, as debility soon makes its appearance, brandy, commenced with early and administered with judgment, becomes an invaluable remedy. Fluid nourishment, given at regular intervals whether the patient wishes it or not, is now recognized as a valuable adjunct in the treatment. The action of all the secretory and excretory organs must be inquired into from day to day, and any irregularity in their functions must be corrected by the use of mild remedies. Frequent sponging the body with vinegar and water cools the skin and adds much to bodily comfort.

There is another disease which occurs sporadically in the cities of this middle region, and may even show itself in scattered localities when induced by specific local causes. I refer to Typhus Fever, which is the pest of armies, occurring wherever animal accumulations are found and known, from its constantly accompanying armies, as the Camp Fever. As its causes are chiefly local emanations which, in spite of rigid cleanliness, cannot be prevented in permanent camps, the difficulties to combat this disease without removal into a healthy region are nearly insurmountable. Hence the frightful mortality which renders this the plague, when it appears among large collections of men. In civil practice debilitating remedies cannot be borne—the stronger reasons for rejecting them in camp medical service. *All prostrating treatment must be sedulously avoided.* Make stimulating tonics the chief dependence, and the best results will be obtained. Quinine may be given from the very commencement of the disease with benefit. Brandy will be constantly required, and when judiciously and regularly administered, will be found a valuable agent. Giving nourishing fluids throughout the attacks, and restoring or correcting secretion with mild medicinal agents will be the proper course to pursue.

CHAPTER II.

Material of Armies Recruiting, Clothing, Food, Encampments, etc.

RECRUITS.—In times of peace an army is formed of recruits, who are enlisted with much care. Each individual before he is received undergoes a critical examination by the recruiting medical officer, who rejects all blemishes as well as those conditions showing a predisposition to disease; the object gained being the selection of a body of men who, from physical and vital perfection of organization, will best resist external morbid influences. Besides, they are men, whose inclinations lead them to pursue a life to which they are in a measure fitted, by the rough, exposed lives which such applicants have previously led.

VOLUNTEERS.—In times of war, especially between contiguous countries, where national animosity rages high, entire communities rush to arms and, with one accord, adopt camp life with its exposures and trials. Among those who take up arms in defence of their rights or for the protection of their homes and families, are found men from every position in life, from those enjoying the most refined and cultivated social privileges, to the street laborer, all having a common cause to support; men of every variety of constitution, temperament and idiosyncrasy, in whom every form of disease is found lurking, ready to show itself upon the slightest provocation. Those who have led lives of ease and luxury are suddenly called up to assist in the stern and laborious duties of the soldier, to share in the common toil and to buffet with the elements. The irregular mode of living to which the majority are totally unaccustomed, is more injurious than other hardships which they daily undergo, to the sanitary influence of which they owe unwittingly much of the health which soldiers enjoy. Exercise in the open air counteracts many of the would-be injurious effects of exposure. It is surprising the physical improvement which the gloved members of high life exhibit, after even a few weeks' campaign, when followed under the most disadvantageous circumstances of inclement weather.

This was well shown among the troops protecting the batteries in the neighborhood of Charleston harbor, prior to the taking of Fort Sumter. When the call to arms was made, the militia—composed in a large measure of clerks, merchants and professional men, most of whom were much more familiar with the duties of the desk than manual labor—with one common impulse rushed to meet the enemy. Many of them of delicate frames and frail constitutions, exposed themselves upon sandy islands, directly upon the sea beach, with little or no protection. They were badily housed, irregularly fed and miserably watered. Their daily duties were with pick and shovel to throw up redoubts, establish batteries and mount heavy ordnance during the day; whilst their nights, when not spent in anxiously watching an expected invasion or performing tedious guard duty during a spell of continuous stormy weather, was forgotten in sweet oblivion upon the wet sand, at times without the shelter of a tent. Notwithstanding, the sanitary condition of the troops was excellent; and many, of delicate frame, returned to their homes, at the expiration of two months, sturdy, robust men, with an addition in some cases of twenty-five pounds weight. All, without exception, were improved by the change of life, under the exhilarating influence of sea air and active exercise.

It has been often noticed that soldiers, taken from the better classes of citizens, go through campaigns of great exposure, with many privations, much better than the heavily-built yeomanry; which can be accounted for in the personal care of the one and the known carelessness of the other. All armies confirm the well-established fact, that raw recruits, in the field, always suffer more than veterans. In the Crimea, thousands of recruits filled the hospitals, *en route*, before arriving at the seat of war. These troops had been selected, indiscriminately, under a pressure. Many of them were young, ill-conditioned, undeveloped in body, unconfirmed in constitution, and hence without stamina or powers of endurance. When compelled to undergo the hardships of a siege, where the strength of full-grown men soon failed, they were very quickly used up. Unaccustomed to either the work, food or exposure, to which they were compelled to submit, they were speedily seized with disease, and when severely attacked they usually died; or if they survived, their convalescence was painfully prolonged, and the least imprudence produced a relapse. An English Crimean surgeon, in speaking of the character of the troops sent to the East, and of the hardships which they submitted to, mentioned to me, that old age, decrepitude, with feeble, bent frames, wrinkled faces and grizzly locks, were seen in youths of two or three and twenty, the effect of two winters' toil, want and misery.

In examining the statistics of the Mexican war, we find this well-established rule confirmed, although the material of which the volunteer force was composed was much superior to the average from conscriptions or forced enlistments. The troops sent out from the States were picked men, well developed in bodily frame and constitution, yet we find a fearful disparity when we compare the mortuary reports of the three arms of the service.

The three classes of troops in the war with Mexico were: the old or standing army, composed of men accustomed to the fatigues and routine of a soldier's life; ten regiments of enlisted men, carefully selected by recruiting surgeons; and 73,000 volunteers, taken at random from all walks of life.* The total loss in the old army, by deaths, discharges, resignations and desertions, exclusive of discharges by expiration of service, was 7,933, in an aggregate force of 15,736; being 50.79 per cent. for the whole service of twenty-six months, or a monthly loss of 1.95 per cent. In the ten new regiments, using the same basis, the total loss was 3,839, in an aggregate strength of 11,186; being 34.22 per cent. for the whole service of fifteen months, or a monthly loss of 2.28 per cent.

*Medical Statistics U. S. Army, 1839 to 1854.

In the regiments and corps of volunteers, the total loss was 20,385, in an aggregate force of 73,260, being 27.82 per cent. for the average period of service of ten months, or a monthly loss of 2.78 per cent. When it is remembered that the old army stood the brunt of all the early engagements, and that many of the volunteer regiments were never in battle, the dangers of camp life to volunteers and raw recruits become more conspicuously evident. The old army sustained a loss of 5.03 per cent. from killed in battle or dying from wounds—a loss of 792 men, from 15,736. The ten new regiments met with a loss of 143, from 11,186, or 1.27 per cent. Whilst the volunteer corps, numbering 73,260, lost in battle and from wounds only 613, or 0.83 per cent., whilst the actual sick list, carefully compiled, and leaving out all losses to the army except from sickness, amount to 15,617, or 26.83 per cent.

These statistics, collected with great care by the late surgeon-general of the United States, portray, in vivid colors, the effect of the exposures and hardships of an active campaign upon those who, for the first time, adopt the life of a soldier. As not only the valuable lives of citizen soldiery, forming morally, socially, pecuniarily, our very best people, should be to the utmost protected, but also, from the enormous expense and trouble incurred by a nation in training and in transporting an army for distant service, it is imperative that the medical staff labor to disseminate among the troops those rules of hygiene which, when considered in its widest sense, are so profitable in sustaining an effective military strength.

We have just seen that in our own wars, as in all that have ever occurred, an army is *rarely* decimated by the fire of an enemy. Those killed in battle are but a handful when compared to the victims of disease. In Mexico, our army of 100,182 men, in an average campaign of seventeen months, exposed to the continued fire of an enemy who contested every inch of ground from the seaboard to their capital, making a firm stand at every strategic point, from which they had to be driven under a murderous fire, lost but 1,549 men in battle and from wounds, all told; whilst 10,986 died in Mexico from disease, besides the hundreds, or I would be well within bounds when I say thousands, who returned home to die among their friends from the effects of diseases contracted in camp. For some time after the war, volunteers formed a noted proportion of the inmates of civil hospitals, and the chronic diseases under which they were laboring were with great difficulty controlled.

In the Crimean service, the statistics collected by Lord Panmure, minister of war, show the English loss to have been 22,457, of which number 3,448 were killed in battle, or died from the effects of wounds received. Whilst the French loss, as reported to his Government by M. Scribe, inspector-general of the French medical service in the Crimea, exhibits the frightful loss by death of 63,000; whilst the admission into hospital numbered 114,668.

The above statistics are sufficient to show that the efficiency of an army does not consist in its great numbers, but in the sanitary condition of the troops.

The duties of the medical staff are paramount, as the nation should look to them as much as to the military leaders for the successful termination of a campaign. Let us now see how this health, which is so valuable to an army, can be preserved.

Recruiting Service.—The first protection which an army has is in the recruiting service, which is a thorough sifting of applicants for admission. The duty of deciding on the efficiency of a recruit depends upon an examination made by a recruiting officer and a military surgeon. The service demands that this examination be thorough, both in regard to moral and physical disabilities. The regulations, therefore, enjoin, that, "in passing a recruit, the medical officer is to examine him stripped, to see that he has free use of all his limbs; that his chest is ample; that his hearing, vision, and speech is perfect; that he has no tumors, ulcerated or extensively cicatrized legs; no rupture or chronic cutaneous affection; that he has not received any contusion or wound of the head that may impair his faculties; that he is not a drunkard, is not subject to convulsions, and has no infectious or other disorder that may unfit him for military service. The surgeon is also required to certify on honor, that the recruit passed by him "is free from all bodily defects and mental infirmity, which would in any way disqualify him from performing the duties of a soldier." As the recruit must be between the age of eighteen and thirty-five years, at least five feet four inches in height, and able-bodied, we can understand why an army selected by a rigid observance of the above regulations, composed of healthy, robust men, in the vigor of manhood, when brought under thorough discipline, is in the best condition to preserve a high standard of health.

To show with what stringency the laws on this subject are observed, we give the recruiting list of the United States Army for 1852. The total number examined were 16,064, of these 13,338 were rejected; 2,726 were alone received into the service. Among the causes of rejection are found the following: Not robust, too slender, unsound, broken-down constitutions, general unfitness, imbecility, unsound mind, epilepsy, intemperance and bad habits, hernia and lax abdominal rings, varicose veins and varicocele, hemorrhoids, syphilis, gonorrhœa, loss of teeth, unequal length of limbs, general and local malformation, contracted chest, spinal curvature, old injuries, fractures, etc.; cicatrices, tumors; diseases of bones, joints, skin, heart, testis, and tunica vaginalis; of arms, eyes, ears, glands, chest, throat and abdomen; defective hearing, speech and vision; ulcers, goitre, ascetes and anasarca, obesity, etc.

When we take into consideration the little disparity of age with the absence of so many predisposing causes of disease, we can readily see why the soldier, by profession, has so great an advantage over the volunteer force, into which any one capable of performing duty is received, however unfitted he may be physically for the toil and privations of camp life.

To obtain the utmost capacity of labor from

men, they must be properly clothed and well fed. These are the pre-requisites, without which their powers of resistance to exposure and excessive exertion are not developed. A soldier is compelled to familiarize himself with many occurrences which experience in actual war shows to be common. He is often called upon for laborious work, to expose himself to wind and rain, heat and cold, to suffer hunger and fatigue, to travel at night as well as during the day, to sleep dressed and accoutred in cloak or blanket. He must be taught when thus exposed to secure his person from disease, and to ward off injurious consequences. In short, he ought to be put in possession of the best remedies for every contingency which may or can happen in military service. This is particularly the case with an armed body who may be called upon at any moment to exert great efforts in making forced marches, and, under many privations, to meet a bold and determined enemy, and to repulse a superior force. The strength of an army is calculated rather by the physique of its men than by numbers, as experience shows that men who have been well taken care of are capable of opposing successfully double the force badly provided. To preserve health and efficiency, troops must be well clothed. This is one of the weighty questions in the economy of an army, and has been the subject of much study and experiment by military leaders.

The object of clothing is to protect the skin from diurnal variations or annual perturbations of the atmosphere, whilst it absorbs excretions, and thus becomes the means which allows man to enlarge his native sphere, and successfully resist extremes of temperature in the torrid or frigid zones. As clothing is the septum placed between the body and the circumambient air, it isolates by retarding the transmission of caloric, and thus protects in proportion to its powers of reflection and conduction. These properties are much modified by the layer of air which is shut in next to the skin, as also by that which permeates the cloth, filling up the meshes of the fabric, this layer of air being known to be a bad conductor. We are acquainted with a familiar application of this law in the bitter coldness of a windy day, when compared with the comfort of much colder but quiet weather. It is the action of these causes which explains why the exterior of the clothing of a soldier, bivouacked without shelter under the clear sky, is colder than the surrounding air. As bad conductors, the heat which escapes from the skin traverses slowly the thickness of clothing, but as soon as it reaches the external surface, it is radiated or emitted rapidly. The protection of a tent or even a cloak counteracts this radiation. The inverse protection which the blanket gives the Spaniard or Arab in hot weather, is similarly accounted for. The radiating properties of wool exceeds its conducting or absorbing powers, and throws off the great heat of the sun before it can penetrate the thickness of clothing and reach the wearer's skin.

Besides the property just enumerated, the hygrometric powers of different fabrics, condensing moisture from the air and absorbing perspiration, are of much importance in the sanitary economy of clothing. In either case their power of conducting heat is increased, and therefore the more moisture they contain in their meshes the colder they are as apparel. The fluid which the cloth imbibes takes the place of air, and becomes a cause of refrigeration by evaporation, robbing the neighboring skin of its heat to form aqueous vapor. Linen, for instance, imbibes at once moisture from any source, and chills the body by the evaporation of this moisture; this material for articles of clothing exposes the body to sensations of cold and dampness, and necessarily to the diseases which are brought on by such exposure.

Cotton fabrics, although not so attractive to moisture, permits absorption and evaporation to a considerable extent. Whilst woollen goods condenses moisture as badly as it conducts heat, from it evaporation goes on very gradually, so as scarcely to chill the external surface of the clothing.

The hygrometric properties of clothing are intimately connected with their action upon the skin, when considered as an organ of absorption and excretion. Cutaneous perspiration varies in quantity, according to the powers of conduction, radiation, and heat-absorbing properties of clothing, which cannot modify the heat exhalation, absorption and sensibility of the skin without reacting upon its functions. The energy of cutaneous elimination regulates in a measure the march of other excretions. Anything which impresses the nerves of the skin excites equally the origin of these nerves, and causes exaltation or depression of the system. Clothing determines the antagonism which exists between animal heat and external temperature. The source of animal heat increases or diminishes its activity according to changes in the atmosphere; but the unequal production of heat causes corresponding oscillations in the movements of respiration and circulation in the action of the muscles and the brain. Clothing affects, then, all the functions of the economy, and may clearly represent the question of health.

As the object of clothing is usefulness and convenience, the best uniform is that which will protect the body from the inclemencies of the weather, and which least impedes the movements which are connected with military duties. Experience in the field teaches what can be dispensed with or what can be added with advantage. The clothing selected depends much upon the habits of a people and the country in which the war is carried on. We can readily understand how absurd it would be in the English Government sending their home troops in their thick red coats, leathered necks and shakoed heads to do field duty on the scorching plains of India. There are certain portions of the clothing which experience shows conducive to health in all countries and under every circumstance. The clothing for troops should be made of wool, whether the material be heavy or light, to suit the climate.

The *soldier's coat* should be a frock fitting loosely, easy over the shoulders, with full play for the arms, without binding in any way, and wide in the body, so as not to impede the expansion of the chest when closely buttoned. The tail of a coat gives much protection to the body and abdomen from damp, whilst a jacket—which is a very poor costume for soldiers—exposes the entire body to drafts and dampness, fruitful causes of bowel complaints. The *trousers* should be of good, heavy woollen material, made also free, for the easy play of the limbs. *Flannel shirts*, coming well down upon the thighs, and drawers of the same material, are of great hygienic utility. In winter they retain the animal heat and support the healthy function of the skin, whilst in summer they absorb more readily the excess of perspiration, which occurs under severe exercise; and whilst agreeable to the wearer, they prevent sudden arrests of perspiration, and are thus a protection against diarrhœa and dysentery, which are so fatal to armies. These should be furnished in sufficient numbers to enable the soldier to change when he has been exposed to rain, as he may thus prevent pneumonias and bronchial affections, so common to camp life.

In the French service, where flannel underclothing is not in that constant use as in the English and American service, every soldier carries a band of flannel, with which he envelops his abdomen, as a safeguard from abdominal affections. Baudens, one of the surgeons-in-chief of the Crimean service, speaks of this band as essential to the health of the troops, and refers to the much better and more convenient protection which the English flannel shirt gives to the men. The liability of losing the flannel girdle, and its very partial protection, is a serious objection to its use. For similar reasons *woollen socks* should always be given to soldiers. They are much more durable than cotton, and much more healthy, preserving an equal temperature and retaining warmth to the feet which, being at the greatest distance from the centre of the circulation, are least capable of resisting cold, and, therefore, require most protection against injury. They also afford a better protection against the chance of blistering than socks of other material.

The feet are part of the person of a soldier so essential for the performance of military duty, that their condition should be particularly attended to by the officers. *The shoes, boots or half-boots* should be well made, of good, durable material, and well fitted to the foot, so as to be easy to the wearer. The soles should be broad, thick and firm, high quartered so as to exclude mud or sand, and closely fitting around the instep, so that tenacious clay cannot easily drag it from the foot. A good shoe or boot adds often as much to the efficiency of the soldier as a good weapon. Marching is as necessary a quality as fighting, and is made one of the requisites in becoming a member of the Imperial Guard of the present French Emperor. When the shoe does not fit the wearer who is compelled to use them, sore feet, a very troublesome complaint in the army, is brought on. In the march men are found lagging behind from lameness, and, as these are exposed to be cut off by marauders, it is the duty of those in authority never to deliver a pair of shoes which have not been tried with care. The leather should be well smeared with grease, oil, wax, tallow or other composition to make them water-proof and soft. This should be done daily in wet weather. In the Crimean service the Russian half-boot was found so superior an article over the boots or shoes of the Allies, that they were sought for with avidity upon the dead as soon as they were shot down, and were more prized than any other article of wearing apparel, so conducive were they to the comfort of the wearer. They protected the feet perfectly from the mud in which the troops lived for months.

The *French gaiter* used in the Crimea, was made of heavy white cloth, covering two-thirds of the foot and extending some distance up the leg, usually over the knee. It facilitates walking, and prevents enlargement of the veins, whilst it protects the limb from cold and wet. Experience in the field and upon the march has proved them so serviceable that the entire French army is provided with them. They, as a substitute for the boot, might be added with advantage to the equipment of the soldier. When made of leather they become hard after getting wet and, by pressure, excoriate the ankles. Beside which, the leather is cold in winter and very hot in summer. The only advantage in the leather gaiter is durability; the cloth wears out much sooner, and also becomes saturated with moisture in very wet weather. In addition to the gaiter, many of the French troops wear greaves made of heavy patent leather, which cover the leg to the knee, shutting in the bottom of the pants. This gives them great facilities in walking, as it protects the leg of the pantaloon from becoming foul with mud, which is an endless annoyance to troops marching in bad weather.

Every soldier should have an *overcoat* of stout cloth, reaching below his knees, with a cape covering the shoulders. This, like all other articles of clothing, should be made easy, to permit of any movements without binding. The French have added a hood, to protect the head and neck in bad weather from cold, wind and rain, which diminishes the frequency of catarrhal affections. When on guard duty in bad weather they are of great utility, and protect the head and neck from the damp ground when sleeping. Crimean soldiers found this addition a great improvement.

In selecting a *color* for a uniform, it should be remembered that light colors absorb less than dark, and also that odoriferous exhalations adhere with much greater pertinacity to dark than to light clothing, which is an item of no small importance when the deleterious emanations accompanying large bodies of men are considered. Beside which, experience in battle shows that certain colors make much better marks to fire at than others; and, according to calculations, a soldier dressed in light cloth is much less liable to be hit than in dark. The following is the proportion: red, twelve; rifle green, seven; brown, six; Austrian bluish gray, five. Red, which is the most attractive and fatal color, is more than twice as much so as gray, which is the least.

The best *military hat* in use is a light, soft felt, with a sufficiently high crown to allow space for air over the brain. The rim can be fastened up in fair weather; and, when turned down, protects, in a measure, from the rain or from the rays of the sun. In a warm climate, the light color of the hat adds much to the comfort of the wearer. The small, jauntily-fitting kelpe is light, but does not protect the face; and, when made of dark materials, concentrates the solar rays upon the head. This can be obviated by adding a Havelock, which consists of a cap cover with a long cape attached, and, hanging down upon the shoulders, protects the neck from the sun in the day and draughts at night. It is made of light cloth, of a light color, for reflecting heat. Those who have worn them on a march, or when exposed to the sun's rays, speak in extravagant terms of the comfort and protection which they give. The advantage of a light and high-crowned hat is, that when exposed to the sun, on a march, a small, wet handkerchief placed in the crown will not only prevent sunstroke, but will add much to the comfort of the soldier.

According to the army regulations of the Confederate service, a soldier is allowed the uniform clothing stated in the following table, or articles thereof of equal value:

CLOTHING.	FOR THREE YEARS.			Total for three years.
	1st.	2d.	3d.	
Cap, complete	2	1	1	4
cover	1	1	1	3
Coat	2	1	1	4
Trousers	3	2	2	7
Flannel shirt	3	3	3	9
Flannel drawers	3	2	2	7
Bootees,* pairs	4	4	4	12
Stockings	4	4	4	12
Leather *stock*	1	.....	.....	1
Great coat	1	.....	.....	1
Stable frock (for mounted men)	1	.....	.....	1
Fatigue overall (for engineers and ordnance)	1	1	1	3
Blanket	1	.....	1	2

In the field, there should be always a supply of clothing at hand, to replace unavoidable accidents. During the Crimean service, Dr. McLeod informs us that the deficiency of clothing, which was so much complained of, was one of the most prolific sources of subsequent disease among the English troops. One of the maxims for preserving health in a campaign is, that *soldiers must protect themselves in summer from night air by warm clothing.* A heavy blanket, not in name, but in weight, and one and a half yards of india-rubber cloth, complete the furnishing of a soldier. The india-rubber cloth is a waterproof covering for him during exposure, and will always make for him a dry bed, upon which he can find health as well as comfort.

*Mounted men may receive *one* pair of "boots" and *two* pair of "bootees," instead of *four* pair of bootees.

We make the following extract, on the extent of a soldier's equipment, from Jackson's Formation, Discipline and Economy of Armies. In the form and fashion of a soldier's equipment, "the adjustment of the kind and quantity of articles termed necessaries is a matter of importance, and as such requires to be well considered. It is demonstrably proved to the conviction of all persons who have served with armies, that superfluous baggage, that is, baggage beyond the narrowest measure of utility, instead of bringing comfort to the possessor, is a cause of great annoyance and vexation. A complete change of the smaller parts of dress, in the event of being wet with rain, together with a cloak as a covering for the night, is all that a soldier requires for his comfort and the preservation of his health; and, as such, it is all that he ought to be permitted to possess. Where persons have not more than one change of raiment, the strong impression of necessity obliges them to prepare for the return of want. Where there is a superfluity, the necessity does not present itself so forcibly, and hence the dirty clothes are crammed into the knapsack, where they accumulate in quantity without obliging the individual to recollect that they are not fit for use until they are washed. It thus often happens that a soldier who has four or more shirts in his possession, has not one fit for use, while a soldier who possesses no more than two has generally one in his knapsack ready for the contingent occasion."

The following is considered to be a full equipment for a soldier on service, namely: two shirts, flannel preferable; two pair of woollen socks; two pair of flannel drawers; two pair of shoes, or one pair of shoes and one of half boots; one pair of gaiters; a small case of needles, thread and buttons for mending clothes; small shoe brush, with blacking; comb and hair brush; one piece of soap; a sponge for washing the body, and a towel for drying it; two pocket handkerchiefs; an overcoat of heavy material, besides his uniform. He should also have a heavy blanket, better if lined with stout osnaburgs to increase its durability and warmth, and two yards of india-rubber cloth to protect him from the weather. He should also carry a knife, fork and spoon, a canteen for drink, and also a canteen or haversack for carrying dressed provisions. If those articles of clothing not in use be put up in a neat and compact manner and enveloped in oiled silk, so as to be secure from wet, and deposited in the knapsack for easy carriage, the soldier will not be incommoded by the bulk or encumbered by the weight; and possessing within himself everything actually necessary for use, will be independent of the accidents so common to the baggage wagons.

In the above list we have purposely omitted shaving apparatus, as every soldier in the field should allow his beard to grow. It protects his throat, and often prevents lung diseases, catarrhal affections, etc. A heavy moustache is known to protect the wearer, to a certain extent, from malarial influences, acting as a sieve to the lungs. It also purifies the atmosphere inhaled, of dust during marches, and thereby prevents many troublesome diseases. Cleanliness dictates that the hair be cut close on the head, and although the beard be allowed to grow, it should also be kept within bounds.

Cleanliness.—Nothing contributes more to preserve health than personal cleanliness; and as the free use of soap is a prophylactic as well as a civilizer, it should be regularly distributed to the men. Daily ablutions should never be omitted; and, if possible, the chest and arms, as well as the face and neck, should be well sponged. Baths should be used whenever opportunity permits. *Keeping the skin clean prevents fevers and bowel complaints in warm climates.* Baudens, in insisting upon cleanliness, says "that the contrast in the sickness and mortality of the English and French camp in the Crimea, can be in a measure attributed to the frequent ablutions of the English, who washed their clothes in hot water, and changed their underclothes twice a week. It is easy to understand how carelessness in this respect will impair the functions of the skin and induce disease. At review, our French soldiers show new clothes, and on the whole an unquestionable military equipment, yet these beautiful battalions leave in their passage a strong smell of barracks not to be mistaken."

It should be the duty of the medical officer to suggest to the commanding officer to insist that these hygienic regulations be rigidly enforced. He is not only the best, but also the most popular officer, who attends himself to the detailed comforts of his men.

Food of the soldier should be plain, nutritious fare, well cooked, which, with exercise as an appetizer, he finds no difficulty in enjoying, however monotonous his daily ration may be. For a working man (and where do men labor more than the soldier in the field?) the diet should be of a mixed character, and food should be of the variety easily cooked. The fundamental rule in the culinary art is boil slowly, and roast quickly. Highly seasoned dishes are neither possible nor desirable for the soldier. Toil, fatigue, and often hunger, will make any wholesome food savory. "The plain repast is sufficient for sustenance; and a plain repast gives all the gratification to the palate of a hungry and thirsty man that a soldier ought to permit himself to receive."*

For the English there is no beverage as tea; and a military writer remarks, that a breakfast of tea with bread, enables a person to sustain the fatigues of war with more energy and endurance than a breakfast of beefsteak and porter. The French prefer coffee, to which they give the highest prophylactic virtue. This is the stimulating drink of the troops, and its free use makes the men much more healthy and cheerful. It is at all times an excellent substitute for alcoholic beverages, which disorganize an army by tempting to drunkenness. Whiskey should only be given out to men on very exposed duty, or in very bad weather, and it is a question whether a cup of hot coffee is not preferable even under these circumstances. The Turks place great reliance on coffee as a preservative against dysentery; and McLeod states as a result of his Crimean experience: "I have no doubt that if the

*Jackson, Economy of Armies.

precaution had been taken to supply the troops every morning with hot coffee, as they went on or returned from duty, much of our mortality might have been avoided."

As roasted and ground coffee has become a fixed article of trade, it would be much better for the troops if it could be served out in this form, particularly when they are upon extra fatigue duty, as it not only saves them much time, but insures the proper preparation of a supporting beverage.

It may be needless to say that good water is even more necessary than good food, and should be obtained at any cost for the use of the troops. There is no one item so prolific in disease as drinking bad water. Should troops be so unfortunate as to be in a place where stagnant or ditch-water has to be used, it can be purified by boiling with a lump of charcoal; after which it should be freely agitated in the air to restore to it the vivifying properties which the heat had driven off.

Fresh meat and vegetables should be served out to troops whenever they can be had, and the best mode of cooking them is in soup. A French military proverb says that "soup makes the soldier." The free use of fresh vegetables is the only mode of preventing the appearance of scurvy among the troops. When these cannot be obtained, the free use of dried vegetables, as rice, potatoes, corn-meal, etc., will tend to sustain health and vigor. In the Crimea, where the temporary absence of fresh vegetables was a great and serious privation, lime juice, citric acid and sour-crout, were extensively used to prevent and to stop scurvy.

Acid fruits are anti-scorbutic, and very good for soldiers. The English, in the Crimea, gave out a ration of lemon juice three times a week, which, when mixed with rum and sugar, made a very nice and healthy drink. This corrective protected, comparatively, the English soldiers from scurvy, whilst with the French it was widely epidemic and very fatal. Vinegar, when freely distributed, also assists in preventing this scourge among troops. Vinegar, molasses and water, when mixed in proper proportions, make a very refreshing and palatable drink, not unlike lemonade, and possessing similar anti-scorbutic properties to lemon juice. A distinguished military surgeon has remarked that 100,000 francs spent in fresh vegetables, will save 500,000 francs from the expenses of sick soldiers entering the hospital, besides the use of the men for active service. Of the dried vegetables, rice is the best for feeding troops. It is easily carried, easily cooked, easily digested, and is the most wholesome of the farinaceous articles, correcting intestinal fluxes. Biscuits, or hard bread, is a common article of diet in camp life, because it is easily preserved and transported. When eaten as dry biscuit, it acts like a sponge in the mouth, exhausting salivary secretion, and, tiring the jaws, it produces surfeit. When possible, and rarely is it not convenient, soak it in tea, coffee or soup; it then makes a very nutritious meal. Even water, with a little salt, makes it much more palatable and nourishing. Fresh bread is always preferable when it can be obtained.

Bacon is, par excellence, the laborers' and soldiers' meat in America, and goes further, by weight, than any other. It never produces surfeit, is always acceptable, very easily cooked, and with its rich juice will make the dryest farinaceous diet savory. It has the very great advantage of keeping for any length of time, under any condition, which makes it far preferable to any other meat for troops.

In the Confederate service the ration consists of three-quarters of a pound of pork or bacon, or one and one-quarter pounds of fresh or salt beef; eighteen ounces of bread or flour, or twelve ounces of biscuit, or one and one-quarter pounds corn meal; and at the rate, to one hundred rations, of eight quarts of peas or beans, or in lieu thereof, ten pounds of rice, six pounds of coffee, twelve pounds sugar; also, four quarts of vinegar. The ration is completed by adding one and one-half pounds of tallow, one and one-quarter pounds adamantine, or one pound sperm candles, four pounds soap, and two quarts salt to one hundred rations. On a campaign, or on marches, or on board transports, the ration of hard bread is one pound.

When the officers of the medical department find anti-scorbutics necessary for the health of the troops, the commanding officer may order issues of fresh vegetables, pickled onions, sour-crout or molasses, with an extra quantity of rice and vinegar; potatoes are usually issued at the rate of one pound per ration, and onions at the rate of three bushels in lieu of one of beans. Occasional issues (extra) of molasses are made—two quarts to one hundred rations; and of dried apples, of from one to one and a half bushels to one hundred rations.

As soldiers are expected to cook their own provisions, and as all are familiar with the fact that as much depends upon the mode of cooking as upon the articles cooked, it would be better to have special cooks in each mess than to allow the soldiers to cook in turn. A division of labor is clearly the preferable plan. Firewood, of course, must be liberally provided, as it is one-half of a soldier's existence.

The entire health of troops depends upon the quality, quantity, variety, and the regularity with which the provisions are supplied. The effective condition and strength of the army, with a diminution of the sick, and consequently a diminution in the hospital expenses, will depend in a great measure upon the commissary department. In 1847 the dearness of provisions doubled the number of sick in the French army, sending one-fifth of the effective regiments into the hospitals. The better paid, select corps, who could increase their supply of nourishment, escaped those diseases which ravaged the common soldier.

Officers and soldiers usually club together into messes, as this living together is not only much more agreeable, but also profitable for all concerned. The following appears to have been compiled by an experienced soldier:

"Officers' messes should consist of the company officers—four persons. The colonel, lieutenant-colonel, major, adjutant and sergeant-major, with the commissary, quartermaster, surgeon, assistant surgeon and chaplain, could easily arrange two messes.

"Messes of privates and non-commissioned officers should number six persons, for obvious reasons, so that the details for guard duty would always leave four in charge of the tent.

"Articles wanted for a mess of six: Two champagne baskets, covered with coarse canvas, with two leather straps with buckles, six tin plates, six tin cups, six knives and forks, six bags for sugar, coffee, salt, etc., to hold from half a gallon to one gallon, one large size camp kettle, one iron pot, one bake oven, one frying pan, one water bucket, one lantern, one coffee mill, six spoons, one tin salt box, one tin pepper box, two butcher knives, two kitchen spoons, two tin dippers, one tea pot, one coffee kettle."

It is always a good rule to accustom an army to adopt the modes of living common to the inhabitants of the country in which the army is found, as certain peculiarities of living naturally adapt themselves to certain climates.

Although war brings with it privations and irregular living, which it is impossible to prevent, the mode of living of a soldier, to a certain extent, should follow a fixed standard. His meals should be equally distributed through the day, and he should never be put to work without having broken his fast, however light the meal be. If this be neglected faintness sometimes ensues, and exertion fails from mere craving of the stomach. In camp soldiers should live with regularity, and the breakfast and dinner hour should be respected.

It is on the march that circumstances prevent the carrying out of rules.

The following is the order which experience has proved to be most useful in the French service. A soldier should never commence a march without having partaken of a repast. A cup of hot coffee with bread soaked in it will sustain a march of some duration. A little meat would be an improvement, which is always saved by the prudent soldier from the previous day's meal. For night marching, an alcoholic drink after the meal will enable him to undergo much more fatigue. Preparatory to marching, the soldier fills his canteen with good water, or what is much more refreshing, weak coffee or tea. The start, especially in summer, should always be at the break of day. After marching three-fourths of an hour, the column stops for twenty minutes. In resuming the march, a halt is made for a few minutes in each hour. In crossing a ford, the men take off their pantaloons, keeping on their shoes. A sentinel guards any fresh-water spring which is met in the march, to prevent soldiers from gorging themselves—a very wise measure, which prevents much sickness.

Water should be always taken in reserve and with precaution. When taken in great quantities it weakens and fatigues the organs of digestion, increases perspiration and enervates the entire system. It is particularly injurious to drink rapidly and freely when heated from exercise, as sudden death is not very rare from this imprudence. The soldier should accustom himself, when thirsty, to drink slowly and in small mouthfuls, keeping the water in the mouth and throat as long as possible. The cravings of thirst are often produced by a parched condition of the lining membrane of the mouth; and by rinsing the mouth frequently, thirst can be allayed to such a degree that but little water will be required, whilst much, hurriedly drunk, will not satisfy the urgent call. In marching, thirst can, in a measure, be prevented by keeping the mouth closed, and in speaking as seldom as possible; otherwise, the dry air, often loaded with dust, will parch the lining membrane of the mouth—a very distressing sensation when it cannot be relieved by drinking. When, during a march or halt, the fatigued and thirsty soldier finds water, instead of rushing to it at once, he should first try and repose himself before drinking; then, having washed out his mouth several times, drink slowly so as to make the smallest possible quantity of water supply his necessities. Washing the face slackens thirst. As good water is not always to be obtained on a march, a soldier should never lose an opportunity to fill his canteen with fresh water. If the canteens be covered with a light colored woollen cover, the water will keep cooler than in bright tin, which absorbs heat more rapidly, and extends it to the contents of the canteen. When troops have had an early start, they should bivouac about ten o'clock in the morning, and lie over for the heat of the day, as soldiers on march should, if possible, be protected from the midday sun. Here they will have time to cook their midday meal, wash their clothes and refresh themselves from their fatigue. This meal consists of coffee and bread, with meat cooked and saved from the preceding day's repast. The want of this precaution, which old soldiers adopt, is severely felt by recruits. The experienced soldier never forgets to keep in reserve a certain proportion of meat or other food, against a deficient distribution or the want of time for properly preparing it. The meal should be taken in the shade, under some protection from the sun. A few branches, properly arranged, will form a comfortable shelter. The main meal of meat, vegetables, etc., should be taken after the evening halt, at the end of the day's march. The officer in charge of the troops should always know the road over which he is to travel the next day, and when he is compelled to bivouac in places where the prospect for getting wood is bad, each soldier should carry on his knapsack a small quantity to cook his mid-day meal with.

In the evening halt, the site selected for the camp, when possible, should be on rising ground, free from low places, and in proximity with water and wood. These rules become of special importance in establishing a camp for even a few days stay. It is prudent to avoid the immediate vicinity of swamps and rivers; the emanations from such are noxious, often pestilential, but fortunately do not extend to a great distance. Interposing a piece of rising ground or woods is, as a general rule, sufficient to turn or break currents from these low places, and protect from their hurtful influence. It would be preferable to camp in the direction of the regular wind currents, so that emanations may be wafted in the contrary direction.

When the halt is only for the night, and the camp wagons with the tents have not come up, the men bivouac under the clear sky, or seek shelter under a few branches, with which they form a rough shed that will protect them from dew. If possible, dry grass or leaves form their bed, and, lying in their great coats and upon their india-rubber cloth, they can enjoy peaceful slumber. If there is no cover for the men, then they build fires, and sleep around these as so many radii of a circle, the feet of the sleepers being nearest to the fire. Singular to say, this kind of rough life does not bring with it disease, as one would suppose. If the men are warmly clad, they enjoy more health when bivouacked than when in camp.

The site of a permanent camp should be dry, with good drainage, the dryness of the soil being tested by digging, to see that a stratum of water does not immediately underlie the crust. In cold, damp countries, the material for tents should be close, and, as nearly as possible, water-proof; and when pitched, a good ditch should be dug around it, with the earth banked up against the tent to keep out the cold and rain, and also to prevent draughts. Communicating ditches should be provided to facilitate drainage. The circular tent offers the best protection against the wind, is least liable to be blown down, and is most useful for winter. The light shelter tent of the French troops, as introduced by Marshal Bugeaud, will be found most convenient for the summer months for an army in the field. The tent is made of the knapsack of the soldier, which, instead of being sewed up, has its sides buttoned together. When unbuttoned, it is a square piece of cloth. When two or four sacks thus spread open are buttoned together, and the centre supported by two sticks three feet long, and the angles staked to the ground by small camp pins, the two or four persons to whom the sacks belong, by thus joining property, have a tent that will keep them from exposure to the sun, and also protect them from rain or dew. This tent is not more than three feet high at its angle. In hot and dry weather, instead of pinning the two ends to the ground, one of them can be hung horizontally to branches of trees, leaving one side open for thorough ventilation, whilst the horizontal portion protects the sleeper from undue exposure. The size of this tent can be increased to any extent by joining stock, as all such sacks are of the same size, with buttons and button holes arranged equidistant. By employing this excellent suggestion, you avoid loading the shoulders of the soldier, or transporting tents for the army, which is often impracticable. In a few minutes after a halt tents are pitched, and the camp has assumed its regular appearance, without waiting for the baggage train. These tents, so convenient and always at hand, were of great service in the Crimea, but particularly in Italy in 1859, where they were the sole protection for the troops.

The *soldier's bed* should never be directly upon the ground; but if beds cannot be obtained, branches or dried leaves or straw should be used, upon which the blankets are spread. This answers the double purpose of keeping the body from the damp ground and also elevating it into a layer of purer air. When the tent is filled, as is usually the case, the exhaled air, loaded with carbonic acid and other impurities, settles to the ground, which persons sleeping upon the soil would be continually inhaling, to their injury. The soldier's bed should be always dry. All moist, decomposing materials, as green grass or leaves, are more injurious than sleeping upon the soil, owing to the gases escaping from their decomposition. True economy would dictate a painted cloth for the floor of the tent, which is useful in preventing the exhalation of moisture from the earth's surface, is convenient, always ready and less expensive than straw. It can be cleaned every day with little trouble, without cost, and requires to be freshly painted only once a year. When straw or hay is used for bedding, it should be renewed as frequently as possible, and the straw should be turned, well beaten and thoroughly aired daily, with exposure to the sun when possible. In the French camp straw is given out every fifteen days; in our army regulations twelve pounds is allowed per month in barracks. As a soldier always sleeps in his clothes, if he has a thick bed of dry straw to lie on, he can cover himself with his blanket; but if otherwise, he should lie on his blanket, well doubled, to protect him from the damp soil, and cover with his overcoat. If he has an india-rubber cloth, he should always lie upon it, as the very best use he can make of it to protect him from disease. It is an excellent substitute for straw in field life, more cleanly and protects better from dampness; it is always at hand and always ready for use. Sheep skins were tried by the French as a substitute for straw They were found to attract moisture and propagate vermin, and were, therefore, rejected. As the tent is always too small for the number which occupy it, they should sleep with their heads as far as possible from each other. In the circular tent they should sleep with their feet toward the vertical axis, and their heads around the periphery, so as to increase to the utmost their respective areas for respiration. After reveille, the tents should be opened, sides thoroughly beaten, straw turned and exposed for several hours.

Extreme cleanliness should prevail within and without the tent. In an encampment the tents should never be crowded, but ample space should be left around each tent for changing its position at least every four days, so as to purify the soil infected by habitation. The earth floor of a tent attracts and absorbs impurities which, unless changed, would soon render it a source of disease. Permanence of camps rapidly induces infection. This frequent changing of tents gives, to be sure, additional trouble to the officers, but this is more than counterbalanced by the health and efficiency of the command. All the garbage of the camp should be thrown at a distance from the tents, and should be buried every evening. The privies for the men are ditches, from three to five feet deep and three feet broad. They should be placed at least one hundred yards from the camps and in an opposite direction to the wind currents, so that offensive odors will be blown away. The slaughter pens should also be placed at a similar distance. Every evening the offal of the day should be covered with three or four inches of earth or a sufficient layer to prevent any smell arising from the day's deposit; and when the trench is two-thirds full it should be closed and another of similar dimensions opened. Where proximity to the water permits, these privies should be established over the water. This will remove a great and common source of infection, which is very difficult to counteract.

In permanent camps, dead animals, horse dung, and all animal refuse, should also be buried, otherwise the stench from them would be very injurious to the health of the troops. But as, notwithstanding the utmost care, in the most salubrious situations, diseases will in time show themselves—from the inevitable accumulation of poisonous materials, resulting from the growing infection of the soil, with its poisonous emanations, from the prolonged sojourn of a large number of men and animals—the camp, unless occupying a position of marked military importance, should be changed for a new situation at some convenient distance. For a permanent camp, board huts are much more comfortable and healthy for troops, whilst for transient halts a shelter composed of branches is much more desirable than tents. Troops bivouacked are always more healthy than those regularly under shelter. It is well known that irregular troops, which act in the advance line of armies, and which have no other shelter from weather than a tree, rarely experience sickness, never at least the sickness which proceeds from contagion, an evil contingent to camps. One great advantage of using huts is, that they are left behind with the infectious air which might have been generated within them, whilst the same contagion is often transported with the tents.

To enliven and relieve the toil and tedium of camp life, amusements are a very necessary portion of the day's duties; and it is found that lively music from the military bands every afternoon will elate the men and remove monotony. In the summer of 1859, during the Italian campaign, I was at Milan when a large body of French troops, returning from the bloody field of Solferino, arrived. In a few minutes their shelter tents were pitched under the shade of the trees on the broad Boulevard which surrounds the city, and the soldiers were allowed to follow the bent of their own inclination. Card-playing, dominoes, fortune-telling, wrestling, and dancing to the discordant tunes of a hand organ, or the sharp notes of an accordeon, appeared to be the order of the day.

Pets in various forms were commonly found

among the troops, and these were guarded with scrupulous care. Many appeared to be adopted by the regiment as comrades, who have been associated together through many a hard-fought field and toilsome march. In the military hospitals of Milan—which were filled with the wounded, from its very near proximity to the battle field and railroad facilities for transportation—it was not unusual to see a soldier nearly exhausted from the tedious dressing of a frightful wound, when he had passed from the hands of the surgeon, take from his bosom a little sparrow, and from the cheerful chirp of this little bird appear to derive much consolation.

Not the least attractive incident connected with the triumphal march of Napoleon's Italian army through Paris, in August, 1859, was the pets accompanying these brave heroes. Here would be seen a goat, evidently proud of its position, marching with military step at the head of a column of ferocious Zouaves; going through the halt and advance by word of command, looking neither to the right or left, as if the success of the day depended upon its military deportment. Here, a regimental dog would show the pleasure with which he participated in this great occasion, whilst the caresses of the company and the pleasant faces with which his presence would always be recognized, show the appreciation of his companionship. These little incidents are introduced to show the longing of all men for objects of affection, and also how many a tedious and otherwise unbearable hour in camp life is pleasantly spent in fostering those fine feelings of the human heart, which keep soldiers accustomed to blood from becoming degraded and brutal.

CHAPTER III.

Hospitals, Regimental and General—Hospital Tents, with Equipment—Number of Attendants allowed—Care necessary in preventing Infection—Value of Fumigation—Female Attendants—Hospital Diet.

The accommodations for the sick form a very important department in the economy of an army, and, as a rule, are never sufficiently ample. With every body of troops, in the field, there are two kinds of hospitals—the regimental and the general. With regular armies, there should always be a third—the convalescent hospital—situated in some salubrious, rural location, where convalescents, by inhaling pure air, and enjoying the pleasures of country life, can rapidly rebuild their shattered constitutions. The regimental hospital is usually under tents, when in the field, if a suitable building in the immediate vicinity of the encampment cannot be obtained.

The tents used as hospitals in the Confederate service are fourteen feet in length, fifteen feet wide, and eleven feet high in the centre, with a wall four-and-a-half feet, and a "fly" of appropriate size. The ridge pole is made in two sections, measuring fourteen feet when joined. On one end of the tent is a lapel, so as to admit of two or more tents being joined or thrown into one, with a continuous covering or roof; such a tent accommodates, comfortably, from eight to ten patients. The following is the allowance of tents for the sick, their attendants and hospital supplies—being accommodation for ten per cent. of the command:

COMMANDS.	HOSPITAL TENTS.	SIBLEY TENTS.	COMMON TENTS.
For one company......	..	1	1
For three companies...	1	1	1
For five companies....	2	1	1
For seven companies...	2	1	1
For ten companies.....	3	1	1

Only those cases which promise to be transient indispositions or acute diseases are retained for treatment in the regimental hospitals. They are temporary structures, to be moved with the army and to be broken up at an hour's notice. They should never, therefore, be encumbered with chronic cases, nor should they ever be permitted to be crowded. As soon as a case threatens to remain longer than eight or ten days in hospital, it should be transferred to the general hospital for treatment.

To ensure a comfortable abode for the sick, the site of the regimental hospital should be selected with much care—the driest spot in the camp should be chosen, and the tent well ditched to give thorough drainage. The floor of the tent should be carpeted with oiled floor-cloth or painted canvas, which will protect the sick from the emanations from the soil, and will prevent the soil from imbibing animal effluvia. It also keeps out all moisture, which is so deleterious to those lying upon the ground. This painted cloth strictly belongs to the hospital tent, and, as an essential part, should never be overlooked. A certain number of bed-sacks also belong to the hospital. When these are filled with straw, they make a much more comfortable bed than straw thrown in heaps, which is the common mode of treating the sick in the field. There is much comfort in appearances, and these beds add much to the neatness as well as cleanliness of the tent. The beds are arranged on either side of the tent, with the heads turned toward the wall. Could the beds be elevated upon boards for six or twelve inches, they would place the sick in a purer atmosphere than when lying on the floor, where the heavy deleterious gases of expiration collect. In good weather ventilation of these tents should always be insisted upon. When the painted floor-cloth is not at hand the earthen floor should be well rammed, and should be daily watered with a milky lime water, as a purifier.

The straw should be changed as often as possible, even twice a week, if it can be procured; whilst, if the patient can get up, the bed should be well beaten and thoroughly aired daily. *Personal cleanliness of the patient is as important as that of the tent.* Ablutions must be freely used, and under-clothing frequently changed. Whenever the patients permit, the tent should be moved once a week, if it be only a few yards from its former position, so as to enclose a fresh piece of soil not contaminated with animal exhalations. This change of location is particularly required whenever any of the low grades of contagious diseases appear within its walls, or cases under treatment take on an asthænic character.

The hospital is allowed a certain number of attendants to attend to the commissary and medical duties of the establishment. Each company has one steward, one nurse, and one cook; for each additional company one nurse is added; and, for commands of over five companies, one additional cook. The surgeon is general superintendent of the hospital. Under his direction the steward takes care of the hospital stores and supplies, and sees that the nurses and cooks perform properly their respective duties. Often, he acts as medical dispenser and apothecary to the regimental hospital. If intelligent, he can readily be instructed in the preparation of prescriptions for the sick, and relieve the surgeon of this trouble.

Not the least important personage in the hospital organization is the sentinel, who guards the door, and sees that neither ingress nor egress is permitted except upon orders from the surgeon. It is only in this way that patients can be prevented from committing imprudences which may cost them their lives. This guard should be constantly furnished to the hospital, and the surgeon is to signify to the commanding officer of the regiment the particular orders which he wishes to be given to the non-commissioned officer commanding it and to the sentries.

Those treated in a tent hospital always convalesce much more rapidly than those collected together in a large hospital building, where, in proportion to the magnitude of the establishment and number of patients, we find the convalescence of the sick prolonged, the number of deaths increased, and the development of the germs of contagious diseases. In concentrating a number of sick under one roof, the laws of hygiene will be violated—it cannot be avoided. Yet, from the very transient nature of regimental hospitals, more permanent institutions for the sick must be established.

The *general hospital*, for the use of a division of the army, is usually located in some town or city contiguous to the army; or, should these be too distant, without facilities of transportation, some buildings are taken possession of near the lines and converted into a hospital. The organization of this, with its surgical staff, its steward, ward-master and nurses, is upon a much grander scale. Ordinarily, the following hospital attendants are allowed: A steward, a ward-master, an orderly (taken from the ranks) to act as nurse for every ten sick, a matron for every twenty, and one cook to every thirty patients. Each nurse is made responsible for cleaning and taking care of ten beds, with the floor and utensils included in the space occupied by the ten beds. His duty includes bringing to the ward and distributing to the patients the daily rations, and also the medicines prescribed at the visit. The cooks and nurses are taken from the ranks, and are returned when no longer required in the hospital. In a general hospital there is always a dispensing officer or apothecary, who prepares the prescriptions of the surgeon and delivers the same to the nurses upon application at the dispensary. In regimental hospitals the surgeon, or his assistant, when present, performs this duty, if an intelligent steward has not been instructed by the surgeon in preparing medical prescriptions. In a large general hospital the steward represents the commissary department. Whoever attends to the pharmaceutical department should be careful to keep all poisonous drugs under key, so that no accident might occur to the inmates of the hospital, whether by design or through mistake.

In this general hospital we have regular wards, which are always objectionable from the number of sick crowded into these compartments. Every bed for a patient should have a certain number of cubic feet, or, as height does not compensate for area, as all the dangerous gases stagnate in the lower strata, it would be better to allow each patient so many square feet, say fifty square feet for each bed. For those who are severely wounded or sick with typhus, twice this area, or one hundred square feet, will not be too much space, if it be desirable to prevent pyæmia, hospital gangrene, erysipelas and other fatal complications from showing themselves. Rooms, with less than ten feet ceiling, are not fit accommodation for the sick. With the constant tendency to a poisoning of the atmosphere from imperfect ventilation, all precautions of cleanliness cannot be too rigidly enforced.

Such a general hospital should, among other things, be liberally furnished with hospital clothing. In European general military hospitals the patient leaves everything behind him when he enters its wards. He receives a bath and is dressed up in the hospital clothes; his own are washed and stowed away, properly labelled by the ward-master. Should he be suffering under any contagious disease, as the itch, typhus fever, etc., his clothing, after being well beaten and washed in boiling water, are fumigated for twenty-four hours in a closed chamber or tent with chlorine gas. With itch patients, sulphur fumigations are substituted for chlorine.

When any low form of disease makes its appearance in a ward, it would be better could it be temporarily abandoned. Then, let it undergo a thorough cleansing and whitewashing, with fumigations of chlorine. Heating the air contained within the closed room by means of stoves, so as to attain a high temperature, may destroy the fomites causing the disease and render the ward again habitable. This course should also be adopted whenever a ward has been occupied by the seriously injured, with extensively suppurating wounds. Should any one enter, at midnight, a ward thus inhabited, the insufferable smell, and the apparent weight of the atmosphere, would at once explain the danger of infective diseases and the necessity for not only constant cleanliness and continued ventilation, but also for purifying the same at intervals. Such rooms, it is said, should be thrown out of use for two weeks after every two months occupation. This is laid down as an important hospital regulation by Stromyer, in his Maxims of Military Surgery, based upon experience and observation during the Schleswig-Holstein war. Chemical disinfectants were not found useful by him when the rooms were occupied; the rooms must be empty. *For occupied rooms, draughts of fresh air are the only good disinfectants.* The slight exposure to catarrhal affections is nothing, when compared to the danger of introducing infectious diseases, by permitting a foul and unrenewed atmosphere to be inhaled by the wounded. It is owing to the advantages of ventilation, that tents are so much better for typhus and severely wounded patients than wards. Pure air, continually renewed, is essential for the cure of typhus. Abundance of fresh air covers a multitude of inconveniences. In the Crimean service, the French attached great importance to the fumigation of their wards. The surgeons of their immense military hospitals thought that they derived decided benefit from adopting the Turkish custom of fumigating with dried sage, which was burnt in the wards three times a day, beside the use of chlorine fumigations morning and evening.

Baudens states that, by using chlorine fumigations at 6, A. M., and at 7, P. M., the dried sage at 7½, A. M., 1, P. M. and 8½, P. M., he succeeded in preventing as well as stopping infectious disorders. A saucer of chloride of lime was also placed under the bed of each typhus patient. It is a question whether these fumigations act from the medicinal virtues which they possess, or upon hygienic principles. The European nations have such a dread of draughts, that a door or window is never left open. We would judge that they were intended to give light, and not air. The only way in which such herb fumigations can be of use is to make the atmosphere so disagreeable that all the windows must be thrown open to get rid of it. As it escapes from these openings, fresh air equally rushes in to purify the room.

This difficulty of ventilation through the windows, which are the proper media for it, is the common subject of complaint among the medical staff of hospitals. Stromyer had to enter into a regular compact with his German patients. He would only allow them to smoke provided they would keep the windows open, using this subterfuge to ventilate the wards. A celebrated English medical lecturer placed the value of fumigations in their true light when he said, "*fumigations are of essential importance; they make such an abominable smell that they compel you to open the windows.*" When these means are used, without affording the impure air means of escape they only act as masks, disguising, by their stronger odors, the offensive and injurious exhalations from the sick. It quiets the anxieties of the nurse without in any way benefiting the patient. It must never be forgotten that many symptoms which are said to belong to a disease, depend upon the circumstances under which it is treated, and many of these can with truth be accredited to bad ventilation; hence the different phases which diseases assume when treated in hospitals or in private practice. If such causes will produce disease (a fact with which every one is familiar), how much more likely are they to modify those already existing. Every physician of experience and observation has seen serious cases of fever, threatening a fatal issue, commence to improve from the moment that the patient was changed from the room in which he had long been lying, with its closed windows and musty smell, to a light, cheerful, well-ventilated chamber. This is always attributed to change of scene, whilst the true cause, change of air, is overlooked.

Typhus cases particularly, should, if possible, be isolated in tents, and ample room be given to each. Over-crowding is certain to produce such a condition of the atmosphere as to heighten the mortality. It also becomes imperative upon those taking care of such infectious diseases to breathe the air as little as they can: live out of the room or tent as much as possible, compatible with the proper attendance upon the sick, and take exercise freely in the open air. The medical attendants upon typhus hospitals, or in such as are infested with pyæmia, gangrene, etc., should frequently change places with those in charge of more healthy institutions; otherwise the permanent medical attendant, inhaling daily this poisoned atmosphere, will be sacrificed to an absence of a regular interchange of stations and duties.

In the best regulated hospitals each typhus case has two beds. Every twelve hours he is changed, and the bedding upon which he has been lying fumigated and well aired. The bed and body linen of such is also changed daily. As typhus is known by its infecting nature and its easy transmission, the hospital wards cannot be protected by too many hygienic regulations. When a hospital has become infected with typhus, pyæmia or hospital gangrene, it is best to close it and turn out all patients. It would be much safer for the sick and wounded to stay in the streets or lie in the fields, than be sent to such an infected establishment. His permit for admission is his death-warrant; whilst combating the elements would give him at least a chance of coming off conqueror. Any temporary, well-ventilated structure—a hut rudely made of rough boards—would be much healthier than gorgeous palaces with gilded chambers, in which death sits in state to receive its victims.

In general hospitals, the blessings of a woman's care, her ever-watchful eye and soothing words, her gentleness and patience, have recently been felt. Florence Nightingale, when she made her disinterested offer to nurse the sick in the Crimea, could have little foreseen the new era dawning for suffering humanity, and the benefits which she was bestowing upon future generations. It is woman's peculiar prerogative, as it is her earthly mission, to give comfort to those in distress; and when the English adopted the custom long prevalent in France, to allow female nurses to minister to the wants of those suffering in military hospitals, the wounded felt that half their solicitude was removed. Now, a sister's care will bathe the sufferer's aching head or offer him the cooling draught to allay his parched thirst; will sympathize with his pains and give sweet consolation to his dejected spirit; and by removing that overpowering weight of loneliness, by which the sick in a foreign land far from home and friends are oppressed, will pave the road to speedy convalescence. A cheerful look, a kind word, a pleasant smile from one of these self-denying sisters, has sent many a thrill of pleasure through a stricken soul. The surgeon sees, at his next visit, the fruit of this pleasantly-administered draught, which perhaps he attributes to his own nauseous drugs.

The experience of the Crimean hospitals, recognizing the vast amount of good which the female nurses accomplished, and the incalculable service which they are capable of performing, when judiciously selected and properly organized, is a sufficient reason why they should be attached to every hospital, and especially in times of war, when their many and peculiar services cannot be dispensed with. To the surgeon, a good, kind, reliable nurse constitutes more than half the treatment of the sick. It is with the most serious cases that their advantages in nursing are best displayed. McLeod, who studied carefully woman's services in the Crimean hospitals, says: "A woman's services in a hospital are invaluable if they were of no further use than to attend to the cooking and the linen departments; to supply 'extras' in the way of little comforts to the worst cases; to see that the medicines and wine ordered are administered at the appointed periods, and to prepare and provide suitable drinks. As to the employment of 'ladies,' I think they are altogether out of place in military hospitals, except as superintendents. As heads of departments, as organizers, as overlookers, 'officers' of the female corps, if you will, they cannot be dispensed with; but for inferior posts, strong, active, respectable *paid* nurses, who have undergone a preliminary training in civil hospitals, should alone be employed. In the camp hospitals, which, with an army in the field, are merely the temporary resting-places of the sick, men should alone be employed as nurses; but in the more fixed hospitals in the rear, the lady superintendents and under-nurses should in my opinion always be added to the regular staff. Their attention should be limited to the bad cases, and they should have the entire control of the linen, medical comforts, and cooking.

"All cleaning should be done by men. There should be a lady superintendent over each division of the hospital, responsible to the surgeon as well as to her own lady chief. Then there should be a store of 'extras' under her charge, distributable on requisition from the medical attendant, and which depôt should be filled up to a certain quantity weekly, the *sister* being held accountable for the contents. Wine and all extras should pass through her hands. She should be responsible for the due performance, by her female subordinates, of their duties, and have a right to interfere with the ward-master, if the cleaning, etc., were not properly attended to by his male corps."

The dieting of patients in a hospital is always

a matter of considerable moment, and one which requires much attention. The surgeon has discretionary powers to order any extras which the patients may need and which the issue of rations does not include. To be enabled to supply these extra articles at the time when they are wanted, and not depend upon the doubts and uncertainties of the regular form through which all such orders now pass—a kind of circumlocution office, where, in time, the articles may be forthcoming—the medical director should be supplied with funds, for the judicious outlay of which he becomes personally responsible. From this fund the wants of the patients can be supplied without delay.

For the very sick, the dietary orders being individual, no difficulty exists in prescribing for them. It is for those drawing ordinary fare, and who require to be guided by some fixed rule, that diet tables are found so useful in diminishing the daily routine duties of the surgeon. This diet list is carefully compiled by the medical directors of the hospital, and contains those articles of diet which would be best suited to the many. As this is a *sine qua non* in a hospital, and gives much trouble in its preparation, I have here introduced, as a guide, a diet table, which might be useful as a basis in preparing one for individual hospital service.

A Scheme of Diet for Patients in the Military Hospital.

FULL DIET.	HALF DIET.	LOW DIET.
Bread, ...1 lb.	Bread, ...1 lb.	Bread, ... ¼ lb.
Beef or Mutton, ..1 lb.	Beef or Mutton, .. ½ lb.	Tea, ... ½ oz.
Potatoes, or } ...1 lb.	Potatoes, or } ...1 lb.	Sugar, ...2 oz.
Beans, or.. } ...4 oz.	Beans, or.. } ...4 oz.	Milk for tea, ...4 oz.
Rice, ... } ...4 oz.	Rice, ... } ...4 oz.	Corn Meal, ...1 lb.
Veget'es for soup, 4 oz.	Veget'es for soup, 4 oz.	Milk, ...1 pt.
Salt, ...1 oz.	Salt, ...1 oz.	....
Tea, or } .... ½ oz.	Tea, ... ½ oz.	....
Coffee, } ....1 oz.	Sugar, ...2 oz.	....
Sugar, ...2 oz.	Milk for tea, ...4 oz.	....
Milk for tea, ...4 oz.	Molasses, ...1 oz.	....
Molasses, ...1 oz.	Corn Meal, ...1 lb.	....
Corn Meal, ...1 lb.	Soup, ... ½ pt.	....
Soup, ...1 pt.	....	....

Veal, Fowls, or Bacon—such quantities, in lieu of beef and mutton, as the medical officer may prescribe.

Wine, Whiskey, Porter or Ale, at the surgeon's discretion.

Two drachms of tea or four of coffee, with one ounce of sugar and one-eighth pint of milk, to be allowed to each patient for one pint of tea or coffee morning and evening.

The beef or mutton for full or half diet is to be made into soup, with vegetables, and one pint of the soup given to each patient, with his proportion of the boiled meat. The vegetables, as rice, potatoes or beans, are frequently changed to give variety to the meal.

The diet would be distributed in the following order:

	FULL.	HALF.	LOW.
BREAKFAST	Bread, ... ⅓ lb.	Bread, ... ⅓ lb.	Bread, ¼ lb.
	Tea or coffee, . 1 pt.	Tea, ... 1 pt.	Tea, .. 1 pt.
	Hominy & molasses	Hominy & molasses	Gruel, ½ pt.
DINNER	Beef or mut'n, 1 lb.	Beef or mut'n, ½ lb.	....
	Soup, ... 1 pt.	Soup, ... 1 pt.	Gruel, 1 pt.
	Bread, ... ⅓ lb.	Bread, ... ⅓ lb.	Milk, .. 1 pt.
	Beans, pot'es or rice	Beans, pot'es or rice	....
SUPPER	Bread, ... ⅓ lb.	Bread, ... ⅓ lb.	Bread, ¼ lb.
	Tea or coffee, . 1 pt.	Tea, ... 1 pt.	Tea, .. 1 pt.
	....	....	Gruel, ½ pt.

The attending surgeon adds what he wishes to the above diet, to suit any individual case in the hospital.

CHAPTER IV.

Medical Service of the Army—The means of transporting the wounded—Medical and Surgical Staff of Armies—The Medical organization in the Prussian service—Sanitary Corps, or litter carriers for transporting the wounded from the field—Duties of the Regimental Surgeons and Assistants in camp and on the battle field—Preparations needed on the eve of a battle—Positions occupied by the Medical Staff during the fight.

The transportation of the sick and wounded of an army is always a matter of difficulty, and is not uncommonly the indirect cause of an increased mortality. The injury inflicted upon a wounded man by a transportation of even a few hours, over bad roads, and in unsuitable vehicles, is incalculable. Wounds which had been doing well prior to the move, take on at once an unhealthy appearance; some slough, erysipelas or mortification shows itself in others, and all feel more or less its malignant, injurious influence, even with the best transports, and under the most favorable circumstances. The jolting of a broken limb for three or four hours over a rough road is indescribable torture. The prostration and exhaustion depicted upon the faces of the wounded after such a transfer, explains at once the problem of why many should die during the transportation, and makes us wonder how so many escape with life, after undergoing such unutterable hardships.

LITTERS.—The common and best means of moving wounded men for short distances is upon litters, which may be prepared in advance, or be an impromptu manufacture. In case of necessity a litter can at once be made from the blanket of a soldier. This is doubled upon itself, a slit being made through the end corners, sufficiently large to admit the barrel of a musket; one musket is passed through the fold of the blanket, another through the slits in the ends, and a litter is ready for use. Soldiers' blankets are at times prepared for this service, by having strong loops sewed to the corners, so that when the blanket is doubled the four loops will come on one straight side; one musket is passed through the four loops, the second through the folded blanket. Where comrades from the ranks are expected to carry off the wounded, this is the only litter which is of service, as any two soldiers are prepared to act as transports, without hampering themselves during the fight with extra baggage.

Such a litter is, however, very defective, as the weight of the patient sags the yielding blanket until it nearly reaches the ground, whilst the muskets are pressed in upon the haunches of the bearers, which renders it impossible for them to proceed with ease or celerity. The proper litter or stretcher is made of strong sacking or canvas, six feet four inches long and two feet wide. A broad hem is taken up on either side, through which passes readily a stout pole, ten feet long. On either side of the litter is an iron rod two feet wide, with rings at the ends, which slip over the poles and form the stretcher, to keep the poles separate, and prevent any sagging of the litter. Two iron projections from these rods, eight to twelve inches in length, will serve as feet for the litter, and will be found very useful in relieving the carriers, as they can then rest themselves when travelling over uneven ground, without the wounded man being annoyed by the irregularities of the surface. A shoulder strap, with a loop on either end to receive the poles, completes an apparatus which is capable of carrying off a wounded man with all the comfort with which his situation admits. A pike head attached to the pole makes it a formidable weapon of defence. Each of those who are expected to transport the wounded is armed with such a pike, and has one iron traverse or stretcher and canvas bottom strapped upon his knapsack. Any two of them meeting together will be enabled in a few minutes to equip an efficient litter. When placed in the litter, the soldier's knapsack is placed under his head as a pillow, and his musket lies alongside of him, or may be hung from the side of the litter by loops placed there for that purpose.

A *framed litter* is one of very questionable utility, as it is a very bulky article, and one easily broken, so that usually, after a long transportation, very few of them are fit for service.

Williamson, in his Notes on the Wounded from the Mutiny in India, published in 1859, has, in the appendix, a plate and description of a *dooley*—a kind of litter used for the conveyance of the sick and wounded in India. In the field service it forms the patient's bed as well as means of conveyance from the time of his being wounded until he is either cured or dies. It consists of a framework resembling a bedstead in miniature, six and a half by two feet, with light posts, which run below the bed six inches. This is slung by two ropes placed on either side from the head and foot, and running up triangularly, the pole upon which the litter is supported passing through the apex of these two triangles. A tarpaulin cover, with side curtains, excludes the sunlight and gives privacy to the wounded. When the bearers arrive at the encampment, they run the dooley into the hospital tent, take out the pole with the tarpaulin covering and curtains, with which they make their tent, leaving the patient comfortably in his bed. These were found to answer admirably in the Crimea, where they were used to a limited extent. This is the most comfortable conveyance for a sick or wounded person, and its introduction generally into the English service has been strongly recommended.

Horse Litters.—Next to hand litters for the transportation of wounded men are horse litters, made three feet wide with poles sixteen feet long. Horses or mules take the place of men, the poles acting as shafts, and supported by back straps or by a saddle with tugs, as in ordinary harness. Each horse litter carries two persons. When the mules are led by men well trained for this duty, transportation by this means is well suited to the comfort of the wounded; but if the muleteers are raw hands, who, holding the mule by the head, attempt to lead it, instead of allowing it to pick its own way, the joltings and sudden jars make this litter anything but a bed of down.

The French use largely what is called a *cacolet*, a kind of arm chair, which is suspended on either side of the saddle upon a mule. It offers a comfortable seat for the wounded, and each mule can carry comfortably two men from the field to the infirmary. In hilly countries, over bad, rough roads, this is found a much better conveyance than vehicles.

The *two and four wheel carriage or ambulance wagons*, which have been adopted in every civilized army, are considered indispensable for field service, and for the transportation of the wounded. The two-wheeled vehicle is the most comfortable. Both two and four are so arranged as to allow of the wounded being carried lying, reclining, and sitting. The omnibus is the most expeditious means of removing those lightly wounded but not able to walk from the field. Where the roads are good, in an open country, this vehicle should not be neglected.

The Confederate service, based upon the army regulations of the United States, allows for every command of less than three companies one two-wheeled transport cart for hospital supplies, and to each company one two-wheeled ambulance carriage. For commands of more than three or less than five companies, two two-wheeled transport carts, and to each company one two-wheeled ambulance carriage. For a battalion of five companies, one four-wheeled ambulance carriage, five two-wheeled and two two-wheeled transport carts; and for each additional company less than ten, one two-wheeled transport cart. For a regiment, two four-wheeled ambulance wagons, ten two-wheeled ambulance wagons, and four two-wheeled transport carts.

MEDICAL SERVICE OF THE ARMY.—The medical service of an army in times of peace is selected with care by an examining board, whose rigid inquiries into the literary and professional attainments, as well as into the moral and physical condition of the applicant, keeps the staff purged of inferior men, and forms a body of scientific investigators whose efficiency will compare favorably with the profession of any country.

During war, the medical department increases *pari passu* with the army. These appointments should be made with a full knowledge of the weighty responsibilities attached to the medical staff, without whose constant solicitude for the health and well-being of the troops committed to their care, the effective strength of an army will be materially reduced. With a view to ensure the most active and efficient treatment of the sick in the army at all times, and particularly during active service, it is not only essential that the medical officers should be men of ability and of high professional qualifications, but that they should possess physical energy adequate to the more arduous duties.

The advantages of having an experienced surgical staff in the field, and the influence which it can exert on the vicissitudes of war, must be acknowledged by every thinking man. Yet medical advice is seldom asked or listened to by those in command, so long as suffering and death are not cruelly felt. The proper understanding between the medical and military staff of an army, with concert of action, will save many a soldier, who would otherwise lose or compromise his life, so valuable to the country in times of need.

In the Confederate service, each regiment of one thousand men has one surgeon and one assistant surgeon. These in times of peace are found scarcely sufficient to attend to the sick, and in times of epidemics or war they are incompetent to offer that assistance which sick and wounded require. Many a life has been sacrificed to procrastination. Upon the first and immediate attention to the wounded on the battle field depends in a great measure the success of treatment; and in any encounter which deserves the name of a battle the wounded must necessarily be neglected by this deficient medical staff. Our experience in the Mexican war proved the inefficiency of our sparse medical corps. European experience confirms the observation that two medical men are not sufficient to take care of the health of a regiment. This was the subject of general comment in the Crimea, where the medical staff were unanimous in the demand for additional medical assistance. In active service, every regiment should have at least one surgeon and two assistant surgeons, these differing only in rank, their duties being similar. Besides the regular regimental surgeons, there should be a medical reserve corps to take charge of military hospitals, whilst regimental officers accompany their commands.

In the *English service*, the medical department is composed of regimental surgeons, with their assistants, staff surgeons of the first and second class, and medical inspectors. The staff surgeons of the first class rank the regimental surgeons, and with their assistants either take charge of military hospitals or act as medical supervisors for a brigade, composed of three or more regiments. The assistant staff surgeon holds the same rank as the regimental surgeon. When many brigades are collected into a division, a staff surgeon of long service is appointed to direct the medical and surgical affairs of the division; and when a large force, consisting of several divisions, with their respective generals and physicians, is brought into the field for actual service, and placed under a general in chief, a medical staff officer, bearing the title of inspector general, is appointed to superintend and concentrate all the movements of the medical department of the army. The medical department takes the military therefore as its model.

In the *French army*, a somewhat similar organization is found. Besides surgeons and assistant surgeons attached to regiments, the military hospital staff, which is a very numerous one, consists of medical inspectors or head surgeons of infirmaries, staff surgeons of the first class, with senior and junior assistants, the number detailed for special hospital duty depending upon the size of the institution and the number of its inmates.

The most thorough medical organization in

Europe belongs to the *Prussian service*, and is composed as follows:

Each battalion of one thousand men has a surgeon and assistant surgeon, who are thoroughly instructed in the duties which they are expected to perform. Besides these, there is to every *corps d'armée* of thirty thousand men, a staff of forty surgeons, who, in time of war, take charge of the general military hospitals opened for the reception of the sick and wounded. This division has also attached to its medical department three infirmary staffs for light field service, composed of eleven surgeons each. These act as a reserve on the battle field, opening field infirmaries which follow the troops and give the first aid and dressing to the wounded. This gives a proportion of nine surgeons to every two thousand men; and, notwithstanding this large number, there are periods when even a larger number of surgeons would not be sufficiently numerous to give proper and immediate assistance to the wounded. In most European armies the dispensing of medicines is performed by apothecaries, who complete the medical organization. In the English and American service the assistant surgeon acts as apothecary.

In recent European campaigns a very important

addition has been made to the surgical service. It is the *sanitary corps or carriers of the wounded.* Heretofore, when men were shot down from the ranks, they were borne to the back by their comrades in arms, who transported them to the field infirmaries, where the surgeons attended to their wounds. Although a most praiseworthy act of devotion to a fallen friend, it was often called for when help could least be spared, as the taking away of so many fighting men from the ranks enfeebles the strength of the command, if it does not break up the corps. It is also well known, that if any from the ranks are drawn from the fight to carry off the wounded, they never return until the fight is over, and thus three are lost to the company instead of the one wounded. Besides, with the very best intentions, these comrades are not instructed how to carry the wounded so that they should suffer least detriment, and the final result cannot be but injurious to the wounded. The sanitary corps, which now forms a very essential part of continental armies, and has been strongly recommended to the English service by the surgical staff of the army, is a regularly organized body, who are taught how to carry wounded men. These practiced hands are under military discipline, with officers whose duty it is to see that the wounded are promptly and carefully removed from the places where they fall to the infirmaries. There are surgeons connected with this sanitary corps to attend to the judicious transportation. They only offer temporary assistance. Should there be fearful hemorrhage they may apply a tourniquet, or show the assistants how to compress, effectually, the bleeding vessel; if a chest wound, they may at once open a vein to prevent the soldier dying in transit. They arrange broken limbs so as to be conveyed with most comfort, and give a dose of morphine when much suffering is felt, but beyond this temporary assistance they never go. This sanitary corps, with litters, ambulance wagons, pack horses, and all other facilities for transporting wounded men, should be in the advance, immediately behind the troops, when the battle is going on. Their post is one of risk as well as of responsibility. Not unfrequently they lose their lives in accomplishing their benevolent tasks. Both humanity, civilization and economy dictate that a similar corps should be appended to every army in the field. When not wanted on the battle field, experience makes them careful nurses upon the wounded.

The following is the course pursued by the Prussian medical corps of a division of thirty thousand men when going into battle: The reserve corps of forty surgeons establish a general hospital at some safe and convenient point, four or five miles from the battle field. Here, all the appliances are concentrated for giving proper attention to the injured. Here, most of the serious and tedious operations are to be performed, under judicious consultation. As this is the resting place from the field, accommodations must be ample, and every facility for treating successfully the seriously wounded must therefore be found, and all hospital stores should be concentrated at this hospital.

Directly behind the line of battle, and movable with it, are placed the light field infirmaries with their special staffs. They are the main stations for medical service, as all the wounded pass through these on their way to the general hospital. At these field infirmaries, the wounded receive the first thorough examination. Many operations deemed imperative are here performed. All wounds are here cleansed, foreign bodies of every kind extracted, hemorrhage controlled, and the first proper dressing applied. As the wounded are brought to this point as they are shot down, their wounds have undergone but little change; the system is still suffering from a certain amount of nervous shock, which makes it the proper time for effecting a thorough examination without giving pain.

In these, as in the general hospital, there is always a division of labor, and each surgeon, knowing his duty, accomplishes the greatest amount of work in his special department. The division always recognized, is the *examiner*, the *operator*, and the *dresser*. Those who are most skilled in these various departments are expected to give the benefit of their skill and experience to the wounded. More importance is placed upon these subdivisions of labor than we would, at first sight, recognize. It is well known that many hands can be efficiently worked by one head, and that when a surgeon of much experience and mature judgment determines what course should be pursued, there are many competent to carry out his suggestions, who were not sufficiently prepared to establish a thorough diagnosis and foresee the probable issue.

The importance of examining a wound as seldom as possible being acknowledged, it is easy to understand why the most proficient surgeons in the service should be appointed, as diagnosticians, to examine, thoroughly, the wounded and determine upon a course of treatment. In gunshot wounds, above all others, the necessity for accurate diagnosis becomes imperative, and this first examination should never be slurred over, however urgent the demands upon the surgeon's time. *Except in very obscure cases, an after-examination should never be made*, as it always gives pain, increases irritability, heightens inflammation and permits air to gain access to the very depth of the wound, which is sure to promote the decomposition of the exudates around the wound, with its suppurative and sloughing sequelæ. *Many a limb and life would be preserved were it possible to limit the examination of the wounded to the battle field.* Let it be remembered that the first examination is always less painful and dangerous than any subsequent one. All surgeons agree upon the success of primary operations, when compared to secondary, after inflammation has set in. How to proceed or what wounds to condemn requires nice discrimination, hence the necessity of devoting the talent and experience of the staff to this very important duty.

In the Prussian service, the regimental surgeons are concentrated in groups with their assistants, rather than follow their respective regiments into the fire. Thus much time is saved and the wounded receive more attention, and keeping them together in this way renders it easy to command medical service when it may be needed for any special, extra duty. This, of course, does not prevent surgeons being sent to various points of the line, to assist the medical portion of the sanitary corps in the proper transportation of the wounded.*

In the same service, the primary dressings for the wounded are carried by each soldier, so that all necessary bandages are on the spot, and no time is lost waiting for the bandage boxes or hospital stores. The general plan adopted by the entire army is as follows: Every soldier carries a small package three inches long and one inch thick, which contains the following articles, viz: two pieces of old, soft, clean linen, nine inches square; a piece of oiled silk or india-rubber tissue, nine inches long by five inches wide; a small ball of lint; a bandage two and a half yards long and two inches in width. One piece of the linen is folded double and rolled tightly over the lint, and over this the piece of oiled silk is rolled, the bandage rolled around this, and the whole enveloped in the second piece of linen and fastened with two pins. This should be put in a particular place in the knapsack, where it can always be found. Should

* Lœffler. Behandlung der Schusswunde; Berlin, 1859.

there be two wounds, the oiled silk and cloth may be divided to make a double dressing, and one piece of cloth may be used by the surgeon as a towel. In this small but very useful package is found the requisite dressings for every gunshot wound. It saves the surgeon the annoyances and delays incidental to the transportation of hospital stores. In the light field infirmaries, nearly all the dressings of the wounded are obtained from this individual package, the very few extra articles needed being furnished from the infirmary supplies.

Stromyer, in his surgical writings on the Schleswig-Holstein war, speaks of the medical department of the army as modelled upon the military. Beside the regimental surgeons, each brigade had a brigade surgeon with three assistants. The larger divisions of the army were equally supplied with superior medical officers and staff. On the battle field the surgeons of the army established infirmaries for the immediate care of the wounded, who were, after the first dressings, sent into the more permanent infirmaries.

In the Confederate service, where so small a surgical staff is recognized, we will be compelled to take advantage of the railroad facilities of transportation, and use the hospitals of those cities contiguous to the scene of encounter, with volunteer surgical aid as our reserve corps. This will not diminish the arduous duties of the regimental surgeons and their assistants, who will find constant employment whilst in camp and on the battle field; in spite of their unceasing efforts, the wounded cannot but be wofully neglected. Modern warfare, in introducing arms of precision, of immensely increased range, and perfected instruments of destruction, has created a new era in military surgery. The conical ball of double weight has become the common missile, and when discharged from a rifle it flies with fearful velocity. Such balls, when traversing soft parts, produce extensive destruction, but seldom bury themselves. Comparatively few of these are to be extracted after a battle. Should they impinge upon a bone, the splitting and crushing is extensive; large spiculæ are driven in every direction, transfixing limbs and even impaling those standing in the neighborhood. In Crimean experience, a serious wound was sometimes inflicted by a large fragment of bone driven from a neighboring soldier. The extensive injury to bones necessitates more frequent amputations and resections. This conical ball seldom fails to take the shortest cut through a cavity or limb, and it has at times been seen to pass through the bodies of two men and lodge in that of a third. Those who compare the dead on recent battle fields with those of former wars are painfully struck with the greater mutilation of the bodies from conical balls. Rarely are they deflected from their course, as is the round ball, which is turned by every little obstacle, and takes up a position at striking variance with any rule of propulsive forces. In steady hands, frightful wounds are produced by the Minié ball, which requires all the resources of surgery to successfully counteract.

Let us now define the duties of a surgeon in the Confederate service, both in camp life and on the battle field.

CAMP DUTIES OF A REGIMENTAL SURGEON.—We have already shown that the fire of an enemy never decimates an opposing army. Disease is the fell destroyer of armies, and stalks at all times through encampments. Where shot has destroyed its hundreds, insidious diseases, with their long train of symptoms and quiet, noiseless progress, sweep away their ten thousands. To keep an army in health is, then, even more important than to cure wounds from the battle fields. But, as surgeons in the service are expected to be skilled in both departments, so that, in either case, the troops under their care should suffer no detriment, they should be thoroughly prepared for the very responsible positions which they fill. Conservative surgery requires much more at the hands of the surgeon than the destructive practice of former times. Every surgeon should now prepare himself for the field, by familiarizing himself with operative surgery. Half knowledge leads into meddling, which is far worse than no surgical assistance. *Many a wounded soldier has felt heavily the busy hand of the willing surgeon who lacked the guiding head.* The surgeon has charge of a number of very valuable lives, and the necessity imposed—by the absence of consulting aid—of deciding the most serious and critical cases upon his own unaided judgment demands, upon his part, self-reliance, which can only be based upon previous preparation. Camp life gives a surgeon much food for thought and ample personal experience, but gives him no time to consult authors and improve himself with books. He does not see so great a variety of diseases as are met with in civil practice, but he has a wider field for observing the influences of external modifying circumstances, as exposure, improper food, imperfect clothing, irregular work, want of cleanliness, and depressing or exhilarating mental influences. The diseases of a soldier, like those of most trades, are peculiar, each trade begetting its own, whilst it gives immunity to others. The greater uniformity in age, constitution, modes of living, exposure to similar external influences, and strict discipline, modify to a considerable extent the diseases of camp. It is especially the crowding together, with the animal emanations from such a number of living beings, that gives character to the phases of disease.

The preservation of the health of the soldier being the sole duty of the military surgeon, he will be expected to use every means within his reach to attain this desirable end, especially by a rigid observance of those forms of discipline and economy which are under the direction and surveillance of the military officers. As diseases will arise among troops, and, as very few of these cannot be arrested by means of art when skilfully applied at an early period, care should be taken that medical skill be promptly resorted to at the very first sign of indisposition. Hygiene must first claim his attention; under the adage, prevention is better than cure. If the troops are about going into camp he must examine the ground and see whether any causes exist for rendering the place insalubrious. When in a friendly country he should seek information from the local physicians, which will not only give him a better insight into the sanitary condition of the point selected, but will also instruct him upon the diseases prevalent in the locality, and the means which local experience and observation have proved most effective in controlling such diseases. He must see that the troops in camp are supplied with dry straw for beds, and that they air the same with their tent daily, so as to ensure a healthy place for repose, and report any neglect to the commanding officer. He must see that the soldiers are properly clothed and well fed with wholesome, nutritious food, and supplied with an abundance of good water, and, from time to time, should suggest to the commanding officer such changes in the diet as will be conducive to the health of the command. If the water is bad, he should study how it can be improved, so as not to act injuriously upon the men. Cleanliness of the encampment and of the tent, with frequent ablutions of the body and clothing of soldiers, should never be absent from his thoughts. He should point out to the commanding officer all nuisances which promise to be detrimental to the health of the corps, and urge their removal, suggesting how they can best be disposed of.

The hospital tents will be pitched upon a dry, well-drained spot, if a building cannot be obtained for the same, and it is the duty of the regimental surgeon to attend to the proper furnishing of the same with all possible conveniences for the sick. He will enforce all proper hospital regulations to promote health and prevent contagion, by ventilation, scrupulous cleanliness, frequent changes of bedding, linen, etc.

At the morning surgeon's call, the sick of the regiment will be conducted to the hospital by the first sergeants of the various companies, who will each hand to the surgeon a list of all the sick of the company, on which the surgeon will state who are to remain or go into hospital; who are to return to quarters as sick or convalescent; what duties the convalescents in quarters are capable of performing; what cases are feigned, and any other information in regard to the sick of the company he may have to communicate to the company commander. He will then distribute the patients in the hospital, see that they are properly provided with comfortable beds; enter in the proper register the name, the case, the disease; and in the diet and prescription book the medicines which the case requires. If his assistant is not present, he prepares the medicines and superintends their administration. He will visit the hospital each day as frequently as the state of the sick may require. Should any soldier be taken suddenly sick, his case is at once reported to the surgeon, who will visit and prescribe for him in his tent, unless the case threaten to be serious, when he should be removed without delay to the hospital.

Convalescents, on coming out of the hospital, are not to be put on duty till the surgeon certifies to the commanding officer that they have perfectly recovered; for which purpose it is the duty of the surgeon to make (daily) a particular inspection of these men at morning parade, to prevent any remaining longer exempt from duty than the state of their health renders absolutely necessary. After the surgeon's call, he will make a morning report of all the sick and disabled to the commanding officer. He also recommends that leave of absence be granted on furlough to those convalescents who will recover more rapidly by change of scene and life.

The senior medical officer of a post, hospital, regiment, or detachment, will make monthly, to the medical director, and quarterly, to the surgeon-general, a report of the sick and wounded, of deaths, and certificates granted for discharge from disability, and transmit to him the same, with a statement of the hospital fund. He will also keep the following records, from which the condensed report to the superior medical officer is drawn, viz: a register of patients; a prescription book; a diet book; a case book; copies of his requisitions; annual returns, and reports of sick and wounded; and an order and letter book, in which will be transcribed all orders and letters relating to his duties. All requisitions for hospital and medical stores must come from the senior surgeon, with the approval of the commanding officer, certifying that the same are necessary for the sick.

The duties of the assistant surgeon are very similar in many respects to those of the surgeon. If he has the confidence of the regimental surgeon, the patients are equally divided between them; he treating a certain number of sick ordinarily without interference from the senior surgeon, except they be serious cases, when he seeks advice from the regimental surgeon. Although this is the common course pursued, it is not so from right, but by sufferance of the senior surgeon. In the army regulations, the senior surgeon being the superior officer, the assistant surgeon is under his control. He is supposed to do merely the medical duties when the surgeon is present—that is to say, making up medicines, seeing that the patients get them at the proper time, apply dressings, bandage fractured limbs, keep the register, diet and prescription books, and assist in compiling the monthly and quarterly returns. When a detachment is sent off on special service, the assistant surgeon accompanies it as medical officer.

When epidemics occur in camp, then the duties of the medical officers become very arduous; the daily and nightly toil which they are compelled to undergo, the fatigue of body and anxiety of mind which is their daily routine, soon breaks them down, and many an over-zealous surgeon becomes a prey to the diseases which his constant efforts are trying to quell in others. This is particularly the case when typhus is raging in camp, when a neglect of those hygienic precautions which the medical officers are instilling into the men causes many a victim in the medical ranks. Under such conditions it becomes as imperatively the duty of the surgeons to take care of themselves as to attend to the sick; for should they needlessly sacrifice their lives, they entail severe suffering on their regiments.

The Crimean surgeons were severely censured, after spending all day in the typhus and cholera hospitals, with tainted atmospheres, for remaining there during the night also, when there was no necessity for it. It was a useless and dangerous imprudence, an exaggeration of duty, which deprives the army of well-informed men, and impairs the utility of the service.

In the Crimea, the surgeons would frequently meet together for scientific conference and for mutual instruction. Here each gave his experience and compared the results of different methods of treatment. Their meetings always terminated in practicing amputations, resections, and the ligation of arteries on the dead subject. The object of this was not only to gain dexterity in the operative manual, but also to find out who were the most skilled and therefore most worthy of being intrusted with important duties. It is said that the mortality of the army amounted to two hundred per day, which gave ample material for such practice. These meetings were presided over by one of the highest staff surgeons or medical directors, who would often deliver to the society practical lectures upon the treatment of gunshot wounds. This plan might be carried out in all armies, as it must redound to the benefit of both surgeons and patients.

DUTIES OF THE SURGEON ON THE BATTLE FIELD.—The common fear which depresses the soldier on the eve of a battle more than any other is not so much death, but the dread of mutilation. Bullets are neither respecters of parts nor persons, and the prospect of losing an eye, an arm or leg makes many a brave man quail before the ordéal through which he is to pass. So that before a battle there is a vague, uneasy restlessness—a foreboding of coming evil, which takes possession of the bravest, and cannot be driven off except by the commencement of the fight. The early booming of cannon braces all for action, all thoughts of fear or self are now discarded, the demon of war rules triumphantly over the assembled host, and suppresses, through thirst for blood and desire for victory, all depressing influences. There is something in the smell of gunpowder which makes men forget their origin; by its magic wand women are made brave, and cowards heroes. In the eagerness of the fray, an intoxication guides all to acts of daring. Who, in his sober moments, would walk up to the mouth of a loaded cannon to which a torch is being applied? Yet on the battle field find the man who, at the word of command, and whilst under the stimulating intoxication from gunpowder, would not face certain destruction!

Fortunate it is that Nature has so constituted us, or the terror of pursuing what duty dictates would be agonizing indeed. The surgeon on the battle field must participate in the dangers, without the stimulation of the conflict; he requires, therefore, a double proportion of courage to sustain him in the trying part which he has to perform.

Upon the eve of a battle, the regimental surgeon has much to do to prepare facilities for the treatment of the wounded. He must see that the hospital stores are brought up with the ammunition wagons, as the articles for treating the wounded and saving the life of comrades are fully as important as those for the destruction of the enemy. He examines his stores, and satisfies himself that nothing which will be required for the wounded has been omitted or forgotten. He examines his instruments, his supply of bandages, lint, india-rubber cloth or oiled or waxed silk, etc.; sees that chloroform and opium, the main support of the wounded, are at hand in sufficient quantity. Water he has not overlooked, as an abundant supply will be needed to meet the incessant, unmitigated thirst of the wounded. He should be well supplied with astringents, of which the per chloride or per sulphate of iron is the best, to control annoying hemorrhage. He should also have a moderate supply of brandy to revive those exhausted from hemorrhage, oil to grease their wounds, and a little tea, sugar, and such medical comforts as will refresh and support the wounded. Having selected from the general stock those articles which he will need, such as all articles for dressing, as lint,* cloth, bandages, oiled silk, sponges, ligatures, adhesive plaster, splints for treating all varieties of fractures, amputating and dressing instruments, with medicines and stimuli, and a full supply of good water. These are carefully put upon a pack mule in two strong iron-bound boxes, called panniers, one hanging on either side of the saddle. One is usually devoted to medicines, the other is used for dressing apparatus. This distribution gives the surgeon

* Carded cotton has been extensively used in military surgery, and was found in the Crimea to be a good substitute for lint by the French surgeons, with whom an abundance of lint is a *sine qua non* in the treatment of wounds. As it can be so easily obtained in any part of the Confederate States, and at so trifling a cost, it promises speedily to usurp the place of the officinal preparation. Now that tents and meshes are scarcely used, and receptacles for collecting pus are denounced in modern surgical practice, we see no reason why carded cotton, with its very soft, elastic fibre, would not make a more soothing dressing than lint, which is often formed of coarse, hard threads, which would leave their marks upon a sensitive, inflamed surface, and therefore must be the unrecognized cause of pain.

Much can also be said of new cloth versus the old linen, of time-honored reputation. Suffice it to say, in this connection, that an army should never clog its movements by an excess of baggage, and that the old linen (which can be used but once) required for an army is no small item. New cloth can be washed a dozen times, if required, which in itself is no mean recommendation.

great facility in moving about the field where his services may be most required, whilst it dispenses with the hospital store wagon, which is altogether too cumbersome to follow light troops in their varied and active movements. In European armies every regiment has such a pannier, which is continually resupplied from the medical store wagons. The commanding general may sometimes have good reasons, under particular circumstances, for ordering the medical wagons to remain behind with the baggage; then the conveyance of all needful medical supplies for the wounded on pack horses becomes imperative.

If the army would adopt those regulations of the Prussian service, which compel every soldier going into battle to carry in his knapsack a small bundle of dressings, prepared according to a formula, then the hospital stores could in a great measure be dispensed with, and with few additions to the individual stock, the wounded could receive careful dressing. The instruments and few medicines which the infirmary would require, could then be readily moved from place to place, following the line as the din of battle recedes from the points where the fight had commenced.

The surgeon should examine the means of transporting the wounded from where they fall to the field infirmary. These should consist of at least two stretchers for every one hundred men engaged, although in European armies, four are allowed to each company, besides light ambulance wagons, spring carts, or any other conveyance of transportation, to accommodate in the proportion of forty persons for every one thousand troops. The character of the transport service will depend upon the character of the country in which the war is carried on. In a level country, wagons are the most serviceable, whilst in hilly localities, litters carried by mules would be the most comfortable transportation for the wounded. In European armies, a distinct body of men are employed for conveying the wounded, so that practiced hands may soothe the agonies of transportation. This is by far the most humane course, and as a mark of civilized warfare should be of universal adoption. It is highly important that a similar body be instructed to act as nurses as well as attend immediately upon the wounded, as this timely assistance may save many lives on the field. In those armies in which this sanitary corps has not yet been introduced, the regimental quartermaster in charge of the pioneers and musicians, form a temporary body of carriers. Besides the litters, each bearer carries a canteen full of water, and the assistant surgeon, who follows the litters and directs the transportation, is accompanied by two men as orderlies. One of these orderlies who habitually follows the medical officer, whether in battle or on the march, carries the hospital knapsack which contains instruments, ligatures, sponges, lint, oiled silk, bandages, tapes, pins, two field tourniquets, a bottle of brandy, and one of laudanum or morphine, or other medicines which may be needed in an emergency on the march or in the field. One of the orderlies is armed to protect the party against stragglers and marauders. The surgeon, for a similar reason, should be also armed with a revolver. The orderlies assist the surgeon in placing the wounded carefully in the wagons; and also following them, are at hand to assist in unloading the wagons at the field infirmary.

When the troops deploy or form for action, the surgeons, with their assistants and pack horses, move a short distance to the rear out of the range of the shot, and they establish their field infirmary. It would be convenient if some house could be used for this temporary hospital.

Where this cannot be had, the shade of trees or the shelter of a hill-side will answer the temporary wants of the surgeon. If the body of troops about entering battle is a large one with an extended line, several of these points should be selected and marked by a suitable yellow flag which designates the spot where those slightly wounded can seek surgical aid. Instead of each regimental surgeon establishing such for his regiment, it would be much better if they would concentrate for individual assistance, when the wounded would receive more attention, and the work of dressing would be much expedited.

When surgeons combine at the field infirmaries, establish at once, if possible, a division of labor; let there be an understanding that those best adapted by experience to undertake certain duties should confine themselves strictly to the same. When each one knows what roll he has to play, and does not interfere with others, a great deal more work can be accomplished than where each one acts independently for himself. The force of this will appear, when it is remembered that all experience shows the medical staff of an army, however numerous, to be always too few on battle days. *Remember that all the wounded must undergo a thorough examination, and all needful operations must be performed within twenty-four hours*, or the wounded suffer from neglect. Now, take into consideration the very small surgical staff of our army and the accuracy of fire of the contestants, with the most approved and destructive arms with very long range, and we will immediately see the necessity of economizing time and labor.

The movements and position of the troops and the character of the ground, must establish the necessity for the greater or less concentration of surgeons at the field infirmaries. As the troops advance, they are followed by the bandsmen or bearers and, if the country permits it, the ambulance wagons, under charge of the quartermaster and assistant surgeon with his orderlies. They station themselves in the rear of the advancing line, where they can distinctly see what happens, and remove immediately, without the range of the shot, those who may fall wounded. It is imperiously demanded, on the score of humanity, that the wounded be removed from the field of battle with as little delay as possible, for early treatment. In gunshot wounds, above all others, early surgical assistance is of the greatest moment for success; and in many, as in chest wounds, what is omitted on the battle field immediately after the injury is received is never made up, with whatsoever diligence and skill the after-treatment is pursued. Therein is the great advantage of having a special transport corps, otherwise the excitement of battle or the eagerness of pursuit carries the line to a distance from the ground where the battle first commenced; and it is only after the victory is achieved that the wounded are thought of by their comrades, who, in scouring the field, find many a dear friend whose life has paid the forfeit of delay.

CHAPTER V.

Treatment of gunshot wounds—What should be done on the field by the assistant surgeon in command of the litters—The treatment at the field infirmary—How wounds should be examined—The character of gunshot wounds—Orifices of entrance and exit—Primary hemorrhage—Natural hæmatosis—Tourniquets but seldom required in surgery—How hemorrhage controlled—Examination of wound for foreign bodies should only be done once, but that thoroughly and as soon as possible after the accident—The history of the case important—Lodging foreign bodies always give trouble even years after injury—Gunshot wounds do not require dilatation—Necessity of examining the pulsations of the main artery below the wound for suspected injury—Ligation of the open mouths of the artery the rule of practice—Water-dressing the only rational treatment of gunshot wounds; its advantages over all other applications—Secondary hemorrhage, how treated—General or constitutional treatment of gunshot wounds.

As a soldier falls or is wounded in battle, he is at once approached by the assistant surgeon, who looks at his wounds, applies the hasty dressing which they require, then placing him comfortably on the litter, attends to his transportation. He can do as much for the wounded in this way as if he were actively engaged in operating. Should his injury permit him to walk, a compress and bandage is placed upon his wounds, if they be severe, and he is directed to the field infirmary. In those with fractured limbs, a rapid glance, quick intelligence, and an inventive turn, at once tells the surgeon what is required and suggests the means of effecting it. With a sword-blade, a ramrod or a bayonet, with a handkerchief or strip of cloth, a fracture apparatus is at once improvised, and the thanks of the wounded, now in comparative comfort, are freely bestowed during his transportation to the infirmary or general hospital. If he has a mangled limb, which hangs by a very small portion of the soft parts, the separation should be at once effected by separating the dangling parts in the mangled tissues. Should he be suffering much pain, which is not usually the case, the surgeon gives him a powder of morphine, with which his pockets are well stored, and at once transports him to the infirmary, where the proper amputation is performed. If the wound be an abdominal one, with protrusion of the intestines, he sees whether the bowel is injured or not. If not injured, returns it carefully within the abdomen, and gives a large dose of morphine to ensure quiet. Should the intestine be cut by the ball, he warns the carriers and assistants from interfering until the wounded man be carefully transported to the infirmary. In case of punctured chest wounds, with internal hemorrhage, coughing of bloody sputa and great oppression in the breathing, the treatment, to be ultimately successful, must commence at once. The surgeon, in placing the wounded man in the litter, will, if the symptoms be urgent, open a vein in his arm to save him from immediate death. To this timely bleeding, on the very spot where the accident has occurred, and not wait until transported to a more convenient place, the life of the soldier often depends. Those wounded in the head, if insensible, require very careful transportation; they should be as little disturbed as possible. Chest wounds, head wounds, and fractured legs give the most trouble, as they require the greatest care in conveying them safely to the designated places for surgical treatment.

It is seen from this rapid sketch that the surgeon who follows the troops into action has nothing to do with amputations, resections, extracting foreign bodies, etc.; these form no portion of his duties. His province is solely to prepare the wounded for successful transportation, and beyond this he should not intrude his attentions. The great perfection of rifled weapons have their influence upon the duties of the field surgeon, as the rapid and frequent changes of the battle field threaten to control, within very narrow limits, field surgery proper and necessitate very hasty dressing.

An eminent military surgeon—Mr. Guthrie—states that bandages, applied on the field of battle, are, in general, so many things wasted, as they become dirty and stiff, and are usually cut away and destroyed without having been really useful. There is much truth in this statement Much of the hasty dressing by the transport surgeon can very well be dispensed with. As he has neither the time, nor is it his duty to examine carefully the wounds, most of the wounded might be sent directly on to the field infirmary without dressing. The dressings, when removed at the field infirmary, are so soiled that they are thrown away. Time, which is so valuable, and also material, which is never in excess, but most frequently deficient, can be saved by adopting this course. Only in cases of sharp hemorrhage would it be necessary to apply compresses and the roller bandage, or what is very rarely required, the tourniquet.

Should the soldier have a large artery wounded, and the hemorrhage be excessive, which is but eldom the case, the surgeon should instruct the orderly, who superintends his transportation, how to make judicious finger pressure. This is much better than the tourniquet, producing much less engorgement of the injured tissues.

Field surgery, properly speaking, commences at the field infirmary. Here all wounds are thoroughly examined, and an accurate diagnosis established. The wounds are here thoroughly cleansed; all foreign bodies which can be are here removed, and the first dressing made. If trivial, they are dressed and the men sent to rejoin their companies.

When the wounds are quite recent, before the tissues become engorged, there is a temporary absence of pain and a relaxation of the injured parts, which favors an examination. The wound should now be examined to its very bottom, to detect the presence of foreign bodies, whether they be balls, wadding, portions of clothing, detached spiculæ of bone, etc. *For this purpose the finger is the proper probe,* and is used on all occasions, with rare exceptions. It is an intelligent instrument, and, appreciating what it feels, it will not only discover the character of foreign bodies complicating the canal, but will avoid increasing the dangers by making new lesions in the depth of the wound. In fresh gunshot wounds, the apertures which the balls now used in warfare make, are large enough to admit the finger when introduced with care. Very rarely is it necessary to dilate a wound, with the probe-pointed bistoury, to assist in its exploration. *The silver probe is a dangerous and deceptive instrument, and should be discarded from the battle field.* Its use on such occasions, for exploring recent wounds, marks the novice.

Balls are readily detected in a fresh wound by placing the patient in the position in which he received the injury, if the direction from which the ball came be known. Portions of clothing and wadding are detected with greater difficulty. Before, however, probing the wound for the detection of foreign bodies, be quite sure that the clothing of the soldier has been perforated. Often a single orifice is seen leading into a limb without exit, which would at once suggest an embedded ball; when an examination of the clothing would show that the ball had driven these into the wound without sufficient force to transfix them, and, on removing, hastily, the clothing, the ball had been extracted by this diverticulum pushed in before it. This examination of the clothing will save much time to the surgeon, and painful, protracted, injurious probing to the wounded. When the shirt or drawers are not torn, no foreign body could have been lodged in the flesh which they were covering. From the nature of fresh wounds, the examination and removal of all foreign bodies will be more easily accomplished at an early period, and with less pain and danger to the wounded; it should be done carefully, thoroughly, and without delay.

A regular report is kept of all the cases dressed at the field infirmary, and a brief description of each case is sent on with the patient to the general hospital; so that if proper officers, in whose judgment the hospital staff can confide, had previously examined thoroughly the wound and sent on their report, no further examination is needed. The pinning a card to the coat of the wounded, upon which is written the history of the wound, saves time, pain and trouble at the regular hospital. *If the surgeon be trustworthy, his diagnosis should be respected, and no further investigation per-*

mitted. Many serious cases can be protected by adopting this simple expedient. In many cases this is the only examination which the wound will need. The neglect or insufficiency of the first examination is often the after-cause of the loss of limb and even life. After-examinations heighten irritation and inflammation in the wound, and, as they permit air (which ought to be rigorously excluded), to pass to the bottom of the wound, this promotes the decomposition of the extravasated fluids and exudations, induces suppuration and sloughing, and predisposes to pyæmia, with its fatal sequelæ. Many a limb and life would be preserved if the examination of gunshot wounds could be limited to the battle field, and military surgery will have attained great perfection when a thorough diagnosis is obtained by this first examination.

The extent and nature of many gunshot wounds are often ascertained at a glance. Touching a limb may be sufficient to indicate to the experienced surgeon the extent and character of the wound and the appropriate treatment; whilst other wounds, which appear trivial, as those in the neighborhood of joints, may require all the skill and scrutiny of the most experienced to obtain a satisfactory diagnosis. No haste should be permitted in this examination to the injury of the wounded through carelessness of diagnosis. Should large arteries be injured, they should be ligated always in situ above and below the point injured, and for this purpose the wound must be enlarged.

As a general rule, torn tissues will reunite, whilst bruised, crushed tissues slough. All wounds in which a probability exists of union by the first intention, should be nicely adjusted by adhesive plaster. The great inconvenience of the ordinary diachylon plaster, which requires heat to make it adhere, must exclude it from field service. The Husband's, or isinglass plaster, is much more easily applied, requires no heat, a little moisture being all that is needed, is not injured by hot weather, and when closing a wound gives as much support as the diachylon. It also excludes, completely, the air, with its injurious influences, which is not its least advantage.

Should a limb be so injured that joints are largely opened into, main blood-vessels and nerves torn through, soft parts extensively lacerated, or a limb flayed, then amputation should follow immediately the condemnation of the limb: field surgery here proves itself the only successful surgery, as all statistics clearly show. If the limb is simply fractured, even if comminuted without injury to the main blood-vessels and nerves, and without complications with joint injuries, they should be considered simple fractures, and dressed as such at the field infirmary. If, in connection with a condemned limb other mortal injuries exist, the impropriety of performing the amputation is clearly seen. When joints are crushed, or the heads of bones perforated, resections are urgently demanded, and should be performed before reaction takes place.

It is, of course, understood, that although wounds might be examined, foreign bodies removed, and the wound, if simple, dressed whilst a soldier is suffering under shock, no serious operation, which would still further depress the nervous powers or cause a further loss of blood, should be performed until extreme depression subsides. Although the nervous shock accompanies the most serious wounds, it may often be met with in the most trivial injuries. It is recognized by the sufferer becoming cold, faint and pale, with the surface bedewed with a cold sweat; the pulse is small and flickering; there is anxiety, mental depression, with at times incoherence of speech. Often this shock is very transient when accompanying simple wounds. A drink of water and a few encouraging words may be sufficient to dispel it. When it persists, even where the injury appears trivial, it forebodes trouble; and a more careful examination may detect a fatal injury. It is the duration, more than the degree of shock, which marks the serious character of the wound; and when this constitutional alarm persists, there is a great fear that hidden mischief is lurking, and the surgeon should be very guarded in his opinion of the case. Keeping the patient warm, in the recumbent posture, with blankets and hot bottles, administering wine, brandy, ammonia, hartshorn to the nostrils, frictions and cataplasms to the extremities is the course pursued to restore nervous energy.

In all painful operations, chloroform should be freely administered to produce the desired anæsthesia. Like all valuable medicinal agents, which when taken in overdoses are poisons, it can remove suffering or destroy life according to its administration. The dangers can be avoided by never pushing its inhalation to stertorous breathing; stop as soon as insensibility is attained. The recent Crimean and Italian wars, in recording the advantages of chloroform in field surgery, show it to be now one of the indispensables for successful practice. It saves the lives of many wounded, who would perish from the shock of a second operation, and also many who would have been considered as without the pale of surgical art, can now, thanks to this invaluable remedy, be benefited by surgery.

In our country, railroads traverse every portion of the States, and as battles usually occur in the immediate neighborhood of thoroughfares between large cities, it is not improbable that they will be found in the immediate vicinity of battle fields. If such be the case, a sufficient number of cars should be kept in readiness for the use of the wounded. Transport wagons are in constant communication with the field infirmaries. As the wounded are attended to, they should not be allowed to accumulate around the infirmary, but be sent off at once to the nearest railroad station, from whence they will be distributed in the towns nearest to the scene of action. General hospitals should have been previously prepared in these localities for the reception of the wounded; and here the regular treatment commences. If it be convenient for the wounded to reach the general hospital within twenty-four hours from the reception of their injuries, many serious cases for operation, such as the resections, might well be deferred from the field infirmaries until the wounded have arrived at the station where that quiet and rest, with medical comforts, which are so necessary for a successful result, can be obtained. When the wounded are brought to the field infirmary, they are not attended to in the order in which they arrive. Those most seriously injured always receive the earliest attention, officers and soldiers awaiting their turn. If the trivial accidents had been dressed upon the field, they could pass directly on toward the railroad or the general hospital, without stopping at the field infirmary.

The common dressings which all wounds receive is a wet cloth covered with a piece of oiled silk or waxed cloth, and secured with a single turn of the roll of bandage. This keeps the wound moist, and is the most soothing, comfortable, efficient and simple dressing which can be devised. By wetting the outer bandage, the cold produced by evaporation is transmitted through to the wound, whilst the oiled silk keeps the parts moist. When oiled or india-rubber cloth cannot be obtained, and no facilities exist for keeping the wound constantly wet, whilst the patient is being transported to the general hospital, a cloth well greased with olive oil is the best substitute for the wet dressings. Many ragged wounds may have their edges paired off and then brought together, with every prospect of speedy union, provided the after treatment with cold dressings is judiciously followed.

It is understood that all those who can be conveniently moved, should be transported at the earliest possible moment to general hospitals, established in contiguous towns. Should there be no facilities for this transportation, then any house in the neighborhood, contiguous to the battle field, must be used as a temporary hospital for the treatment of those seriously wounded, whose safety depends upon absolute quiet, rest and careful nursing; or tents can be pitched for the temporary accommodation of the wounded. Should the army advance, the regimental surgeons must follow their commands, leaving either an assistant or an extra medical attendant for the wounded, it being presumed that a reserve medical corps had been attached to the army for extra or reserved duty, when it was known at head-quarters that a battle was expected. These reserve surgeons will make every preparation for the comfort and accommodation of the wounded. Should the army unfortunately meet with a reverse, all available transport must be pressed into the service for the removal of the wounded to the rear, and they must be sent off as speedily as possible. If this had been attended to from the commencement of the engagement, there would be fewer to move later in the day, when a retreat was compulsory. No wounded soldier, whose injuries are so slight that he can walk, should ever be carried, as he takes up a place in the transport wagon which excludes one who cannot assist himself.

There are many cases of injury to which long transportation would be certain death. If the general hospital cannot be conveniently reached, such cases must be treated at some farm-house contiguous to the field of battle; and if troops are compelled to retreat, humanity dictates that the severely wounded should always be left to the enemy, with a sufficient number of competent surgeons to look after their wants. When left without surgeons, they are always neglected, and many lives may be sacrificed for want of that immediate attention which the enemy's surgeons must first give to their own wounded, and which precious time can never be recovered. This becomes especially urgent where the nations at war speak different languages. The rule now recognized in civilized warfare is, always to leave competent surgeons with the wounded who are left to be cared for by the enemy.

Appearance of Gunshot Wounds.—We have

already stated that the more perfect and destructive arms now in use in modern warfare, and the variety, form and size of missiles, have modified materially the symptoms and march of gunshot wounds. The conical shot, with its excessive momentum, transfixes the tissues with great rapidity, and when only soft parts are involved, the crushing and bruising is by no means so extensive as with round ball. The entrance made by a conical ball in the skin is oval and sometimes even linear, as if made by the point of a sabre. Usually, they pass directly through the soft parts, rarely burying themselves, and, when not impeded in their transit, there is but little difference between the two orifices of entrance and exit. When the conical ball, entering point foremost, and meeting some resistance in its course through the tissues, is either changed in form or is turned upon its side, the orifice of exit is found very large, irregularly torn, with the surrounding tissues much bruised.

Round balls usually give an entrance surrounded by blackened, inverted tissues; these having been evidently mashed or crushed by the ball prior to its entrance. The orifice of exit is usually more or less everted and lacerated. These two orifices are, however, modified in appearance by so many circumstances—the form, size, velocity and number of the missiles; changes in the missile after its entrance into the body and prior to its escape; the distance of the wounded party, his position, his clothing, foreign bodies which may have been about his person, and driven before the ball, etc.—that in some cases, without the history of the accident from the patient or those who saw the occurrence, it would be difficult to determine which opening was first made.

The effects produced by the action of the ball upon the two orifices can be easily understood when it is remembered that in entering, the tissues, which are being perforated, are supported by the entire thickness of limb, so that often the ball carries before it a piece of flesh which it has cut out as by a die, and hence the more or less rounded appearance of this opening; whilst after traversing the limb in making its exit, the tissues through which it is now pushing have no support, they are stretched inordinately before they are torn, hence the flap-like lacerations of this exit, with sometimes nothing more than a rent or split in the skin. All who are familiar with the driving of a nail through a board or firing at the same with a pistol, will see a rough working of this principle.

These peculiarities are said to be so stamped upon the clothing, that often, by an examination of them alone, a diagnosis can be established.

It is often of consequence to determine the character of these apertures, so as to distinguish between a traversed ball, with its two orifices, or two balls embedded. At the same time it must not be forgotten that one ball may make several openings, by the ball being divided in the limb upon a sharp crest of bone. Such cases are not unusual where the round musket ball strikes. A half of the ball may pass out, a portion remaining behind. A single ball, by splitting in this way against some obstacle in the flesh, has been known to break into six pieces, each in exit making a corresponding wound.

Conical balls show much less deviation than round balls. They usually follow a straight course, ploughing through all opposing structures: nothing resists the penetrating force of these projectiles. They seldom follow the contour of bones, as do often the round, but at once crush them; their double weight and increased velocity making many more fractures than the round ball of former wars.

In spite of the rapid passage of even conical

balls, some of the tissues, through their toughness and elasticity, escape direct injury from them. Arteries come under this head. Owing to their peculiar structure, cylindrical form and loose connections, lying on a bed of very loose cellular tissue, which permits of considerable movement, they often escape transfixion, when their position lies evidently in the direct course of the ball. From the battle fields of Italy, I saw several of the wounded in the hospitals at Milan, who had received such injuries about the root of the neck, where balls had traversed in some cases, antero-posteriorily, in others laterally, going deeply through the soft parts, yet picking their way, as it were with such care, as to avoid the great vessels among which the missile had channeled its course. So great is this power of avoiding perforation in the large arteries, that rarely does death take place on the battle field from division of the large vessels of the extremities by bullets. When a ball strikes a limb fairly, at right angles, it produces the least injury to the tissue which it traverses; it forms a simple canal, which might heal with very little suppuration or sloughing: but when it strikes at an angle, particularly when the ball has lost a part of its momentum, it ploughs up the tissues frightfully, and extensive destruction follows.

Although cases are upon record where gunshot wounds have healed by the first intention, the surgeon must not look for such a happy result. With but rare exceptions, suppuration is the rule, and he must be prepared to control its action, and the excessive reaction which, in most cases, would accompany it.

A certain amount of hemorrhage always accompanies gunshot wounds; but owing to the irregularity and the asperities of the sides of the wound favoring the clotting of blood, we usually find that the external escape soon ceases, whilst internal hemorrhage, to a limited extent, extravasates into the surrounding tissues. When the divided blood-vessels are so closed that the blood-cells can no longer escape, serous oozing still goes on infiltrating the tissues. These are the causes of the rapid swelling which follows gunshot wounds.

The pain which accompanies the reception of gunshot injuries is often so trivial, that the attention of the wounded is only called to the fact by blood streaming down his legs. The majority liken the striking of a ball to a smart blow with a supple walking cane, whilst with a few the pain is very severe, and simulates the feeling which would be produced by running a red-hot wire through the flesh. McLeod mentions the case of an officer who had both of his legs carried away, and who only became aware of the injury which he had received when he attempted to rise.

It appears as if every gunshot wound was accompanied by a certain amount of shock, or a partial paralysis of sensation, which is nature's preparation, permitting a thorough examination, with little or no pain. The unusual quiet of a hospital the night following a battle has been repeatedly noticed, and is accounted for by this nervous shock. When this condition passes off, then reaction brings with it much suffering. In this nervous shock, with the suspension of activity in the circulatory function, lies the safety of many a wounded soldier. Its influence is immediately felt in the injured tissues, and the infiltration and engorgement of these are prevented. When nervous depression exists, but little blood escapes from the injured vessels, and as there is no force from behind, owing to the diminished action of the heart, to drive on and keep in motion this blood, its clotting is favored. When reaction ensues, the clot is already so firmly established that it cannot be displaced; the injured vessels remain thoroughly and permanently plugged up, and the dangers from immediate hemorrhage are prevented.

As the wounded soldier is always clamorous of having his injuries attended to as early as possible, and as experience teaches, that all wounds, and above all others gunshot wounds, are benefited by immediate dressing, they should be attended to on the field of battle; then they give less trouble to the surgeon, less pain to the soldier, and much better final results in treatment. Here all hasty dressings or examinations are to be deprecated, and a methodical course pursued. The indications of treatment, in all gunshot wounds, are, 1st, To control hemorrhage; 2d, To cleanse the wound by removing all foreign bodies, and, 3d, To apply such dressings and pursue such a rational course of treatment as will establish rapid cicatrization.

Hemorrhage, which produces such terror in the bystanders and anxiety in the patient, should never unnerve the surgeon, who requires all of his self-possession and surgical tact to cope successfully with this ebbing away of life. Fortunately, in gunshot wounds, serious hemorrhage is of rare occurrence; and when the largest arteries are injured, they either cease bleeding spontaneously, or the patient dies so rapidly, that art is of little avail. If the case is not injuriously interfered with, the natural hemostatics soon controls the bleeding. The ragged character of the wound, and the nervous shock accompanying the injury, or brought on by the loss of blood, reacting upon the circulatory organs, so diminishes the heart's impulse and drives so little blood to the extremities, as to favor a stagnation of blood in the wound. The formation of a clot plugs up the orifice in a bleeding vessel, and stops any further loss of blood.

This spontaneous arrest of hemorrhage is usually permanent; and if the ordinary prophylactic course is pursued of absolute rest and quiet, with the limb elevated and bandaged, no return shows itself. Should, on the contrary, meddlesome surgery suggest the use of a tourniquet, which cuts off the circulation and especially the veinous return, the limb soon swells, tissues become engorged, excessive extravasation in the wound follows, and a train is laid for future mischief. The field tourniquet, in former days, was so much in vogue that it was considered indispensable on the battle field, and was therefore carried in large numbers, to be applied to every limb from which blood was trickling, or from which hemorrhage was feared. Now, they are nearly discarded from field service, and recent experience recommends their abolition from the field, as doing more harm than good to the wounded. Unless very tightly applied, it is of no service, as it does not control the bleeding, and if firmly applied it acts as a general ligature around the extremity, and can be used but for a short time without injury to the limb.

Recent writers warn surgeons of the too hasty use of hemostatics, and suggest that it is better for the wounded to lose a little blood, which will diminish the heart's propulsive force, than have the wounded tissues filled with extravasated blood. If the hemorrhage be free, immediately after the receipt of injury, the best mode of controlling it would be the application of a ball of lint, a compress, or sponge over the wound, secured by a bandage, which, in closing the outer orifice, favors the formation of a clot. If the hemorrhage is at all active, as if from some large artery, in addition to the compress on the wound, the entire limb should be carefully enveloped in a bandage, to some distance above the injury, so that by compressing the soft parts it could diminish the amount of circulating fluid in the limb, and prevent the ingress of blood into the tissues. The hemostatic properties of this dressing can be increased by soaking the sponge or compress covering the wound with the per chloride or per sulphate of iron, which, as a powerful astringent, when coming in contact with fresh blood, will immediately form a clot. A lump of ice placed upon the compress will act with equal efficiency. A sponge or compress, with or without the iron styptic, tied on the bleeding wound, is all that the surgeon superintending the transportation of the wounded is expected to do. Unless the hemorrhage is very violent, threatening immediate destruction of life, the tourniquet is rarely required. All recent writers on military surgery recommend that field tourniquets be dispensed with, as they are generally a useless, and often when carelessly used, a dangerous instrument. The finger pressure of an intelligent assistant is better than any tourniquet ever made, and is a far preferable means of controlling excessive hemorrhage, which the compress and bandage may fail to check. The femoral artery, for any injury to its trunk or large branches, should be compressed in the groin where it runs over the pubic bone; the brachial, where it pulsates against the head of the humerus, as here its course is nearly subcutaneous.

When the position of these main trunks are shown to any intelligent assistant, and he is made to recognize the throbbing of the artery, he will have no difficulty in keeping the vessel compressed during the transportation.

As soon as the wounded arrives at the temporary resting place where the surgeons are assembled, all bandages are removed, and the wound carefully examined. A glance at the wound when the clothing has been previously examined, will often tell when there are two orifices differing in appearance and in a direct line with each other, whether foreign bodies have lodged or not. As the patient is now faint from loss of blood and from nervous depression, the wound not yet being painful or swollen, the *surgeon using his finger, which is the only admissible probe on such occasions that the military surgeon of experience recognizes*, examines the entire extent of the wound, searching for foreign bodies.

This examination is made without fear of reproducing hemorrhage, as the finger cannot displace the clots which hold firmly to the openings in the vessels. Every surgeon has noticed how rudely a stump might be sponged, and what force it requires to wipe away clots which have formed over the face of a smooth, incised, open wound.

The adhesions are increased a hundred-fold by the irregularities of a concealed bullet track. The finger finds no difficulty in entering a hole through which a bullet has passed, if examined, as every wound should be, before swelling has taken place.

A silver probe will travel in the direction given to it by the surgeon, in examining fresh wounds, and *as most persons guide the probe instead of allowing the probe to guide them*, the true course of a ball can only be determined by it with great difficulty. It is but recently that I saw a physician of experience, in seeking the course of a ball which had lodged in the thigh, apparently without effort, pass the probe among the muscles quite across the limb; so that, the bullet wound being on the outer side of the thigh, the end of the probe could be felt under the skin on its inner side. When the finger was introduced it followed the track of the ball at a very oblique course from the one which the probe had taken. This example is sufficient to show why military surgeons denounce the silver probe, and distinguish by its use the tyro in surgical practice.

The wound is examined from both sides, with the double object of finding foreign bodies which may have lodged, and seeing the proximity of the course of the ball to the main arteries of the limb. It is a matter of great importance to determine the condition of large vessels, whether they be injured or not, by examining the degree of pulsation which they possess; as an injury would necessitate a very careful after-treatment to avoid secondary hemorrhage.

Should but one opening exist, and all the clothes of the soldier covering the wound be torn, the probability is, that foreign bodies complicate the wound. It must be remembered that the ball as a hard body can usually be readily recognized, but that portions of wadding or clothing may be readily mistaken for a clot of blood or the ragged lining of the wound. This is particularly the case when they become saturated with the secretions. Forewarned being forearmed, the surgeon, remembering these difficulties, will examine with special care for these soft, foreign complications. When found they should be extracted, as their presence is certain to establish a high degree of inflammatory excitement, with profuse subsequent suppuration.

This effect was well shown in the case of a private of the 2d Regiment of South Carolina Volunteers, who, during the attack on Fort Sumter, was shot by the accidental discharge of a musket.

The ball entered the chest at the anterior fold of the armpit, fractured the clavicle, and after a course of nearly six inches, was stopped by the tough skin over the posterior portion of the shoulder. The ball was readily detected by the regimental surgeon, and, by an incision through the skin, was easily removed. Inflammation of a high grade followed. He was sent up to a city hospital one week after the accident, when he was losing from three to four ounces of pus daily from the wound. On the day after his admission, in examining the wound, I detected in the shoulder wound some substance resembling a slough, and upon extracting it, found a mass of wadding over two inches long and as thick as the finger, which tent-like mass had been driven into the tissues by the ball. Examination of his clothing now, for the first time, showed the deficiency in the lining of his coat from which this mass had been torn. The removal of this irritant diminished the discharge immediately, so that, in the succeeding twenty-four hours, the discharge diminished to one-sixth its former quantity, and in four days was hardly sufficient to soil the dressing.

The history of the case is of much importance in examining wounds. Often, the course of the ball cannot be discovered without it. What surgeon, however great his experience, seeing a wound made in the arm by a ball, would think of looking in the opposite thigh for its place of lodgment, did he not learn that the injury was received from above, whilst mounting a scaling-ladder, with arms raised above the patient's head? The ball entering the back of the arm near the elbow, passed down the arm under the shoulder-blade, across the loin and, traversing the buttock, lodged under the skin of the outer part of the opposite thigh, where it was found, and removed. Knowing the direction from whence the ball came, and the position in which the soldier was placed, you know at once the course which the ball most probably took; and your examinations in that direction will not only save much time, but save the patient much suffering and annoyance. Often, the play of a muscle will shut off the track of the ball. The relations of the soft parts vary with every position of the limb, and a passage made when a limb was flexed, could not be followed when the same limb is extended. Hence the necessity of placing the limb in the same position in which it was when the injury was received.

The wound having been carefully examined

by the finger within and careful manipulations without, and the foreign body detected, it should be at once removed. This rule may nearly be considered absolute, as all military surgeons place great weight upon its accomplishment. The question is not so much whether balls *can* remain innocuous in the flesh, *but do they?* Those who have had experience in gunshot wounds in the field, know how excessive is the irritability caused by the presence of a ball in a wound; how restless and irritable the patient is until it is removed; how profuse the suppuration and prolonged the period of treatment in those cases in which it has been left; and how frequently the after-consequences are so distressing, the pain so permanent, and discharge so constant, as to demand future interference or make life a burden. If such be the case with ball, how much the more urgent the extraction of the foreign bodies is indicated, especially fragments of shell, portions of clothing, etc.

Balls may, in time, become encysted, but these are exceptional cases; and even when such occur, their presence in after years may set up inflammation, which will mat together and bind down important parts, whose usefulness depends upon freedom of motion. Repeated abscesses may form, pressure upon bones may give rise to ulceration and a tedious exfoliation, blood-vessels may ulcerate, nerves be painfully compressed, and life rendered miserable, if not jeopardized.

In McLeod's Surgery of the Crimea, the report of M. Hutin, chief surgeon of the Hotel des Invalides, is given, which is a striking commentary in favor of the removal of all foreign bodies. He reports that of 4,000 cases examined by him, in which balls had remained unremoved, only twelve men suffered no inconvenience; and the wounds of two hundred continued to open and close continually till the foreign body was removed.

If the ball be felt loose in the soft parts, a bullet forceps can be made to seize it; and it can be extracted without difficulty, *provided the disengaged hand of the surgeon support the limb on the opposite side to that at which the forceps is introduced.* Otherwise the ball glides in front of the forceps and cannot be seized. The ordinary bullet forceps, as simulating the dressing forceps of the pocket case, was the instrument preferred by Larrey, and is still, deservedly, in general use. Many changes have been made in these, without advancing to any extent the merits of the instrument. A very good bullet forceps is one terminating with a sharp prong on either blade, at right angles to the blade, so that when closed the points are protected by the blades. These act as an axis upon which the ball may be rolled out of the wound, instead of being drawn out as with the dressing forceps.

When a ball is firmly imbedded in bone, it is removed by boring into it with a gimlet, which holds it securely and permits sufficient force being used for dislodging it, or it may be cut out by using a trephine. Should a ball have traversed a limb, as it often does, and its escape be resisted by the tough, elastic skin which very often successfully impedes the further progress of the ball, it should be removed by making an incision over its position, and not be sought and drawn through the entire length of track which it had traversed.

Baudens, in noting the difficulty of extracting these subcutaneous balls, ascribes it to a layer of cellular tissue, which firmly and completely caps the ball. It is thin enough to be diaphinous, and yet tough enough to clasp and hold firmly the bullet. Guthrie speaks of the difficulties of extraction depending upon the surgeon being too fearful of increasing the incision. Balls can be extracted with the least pain and with great rapidity by making a bold incision. This course marks the difference between civil and military surgery; half an inch added to the incision does not increase its dangers, and expedites the extraction. Be quite sure, however, that you are cutting upon a ball and not upon some bony prominence, which comparison with the opposite limb should warn you from. It is sufficient to mention that such mistakes have happened to military surgeons.

By foreign bodies we mean balls, pieces of clothing, spiculæ of bone, which have been broken off and are loose in the wound, and any articles about the person which may have been driven before the ball. These should all be removed immediately after the injury has been received, and before swelling or infiltration renders the task difficult. When done early, the wound will be found sufficiently large to allow of the easy extraction without dilating. It is only when this early attention is neglected, and the wound has closed by inflammatory effusions, that the removal is painful and difficult, requiring, in some instances, the use of the knife to enlarge the passage.

The dilatation of gunshot wounds, which was

formerly the constant rule of practice, is now altogether rejected from military surgery, unless it be for the special purpose of ligating a bleeding artery, or extracting a foreign body which, from changes in the wound, cannot be readily extracted without injury to the soft parts. This old medical dogma was based neither upon experience nor observation, and is now very properly considered useless, injurious and barbarous. When a ball alone complicates a wound, if it be not readily found, after a careful and intelligent search, rather than continue the examination from day to day, which can only be prejudicial to the case, from the irritation and inflammation which will be excited, it would save the surgeon much anxiety and the patient much annoyance, if the ball or other foreign body be left until suppuration be well established. Then it will gradually expose its situation, and can be much more readily removed than during the height of reaction when the parts are very much swollen and very painful. The surgeon will assist nature in the expulsion as soon as the swelling has subsided to such an extent that the finger or instrument can again be introduced into the wound.

The above rules apply chiefly to gunshot wounds of the extremities; those of the trunk and head offer so many exceptions to the above, and require, in a measure, such special treatment, that the course to be pursued in these wounds, complicated with foreign bodies, will be specially dealt with in discussing special injuries.

We have already stated that fatal hemorrhage, from the large vessels of the extremities, rarely occurs on the battle field, and that when the large arteries are wounded, the hemorrhage is either so immediately fatal that no assistance can be rendered, or it ceases spontaneously. The nervous depression so common to shot wounds with its tendency to syncope, and its control over the circulatory organs, checks the impulse and supply of blood through the injured vessel, and promotes the formation of clots. Openings in arteries may be closed by foreign bodies, and in such cases hemorrhage would recur when these are extracted. The largest arteries may however, be wounded, and may cease bleeding spontaneously.

The only means of detecting this injury would be in examining carefully the strength of pulsation in the vessel, beyond the course of injury. A diminution of its force, when compared to that of the corresponding vessel in the opposite limb, shows conclusively some hindrance to the circulation. When no external hemorrhage exists, an absence of pulsation in the course of the artery below the wound is the only means of detecting serious injury to the vessel, and it often decides whether the limb should be at once amputated. The presence of the pulse is, of course, no indication that no injury has been received. Although, from the course of the ball and the flow of blood, we know that the main vessel of the limb has been injured, if the bleeding has ceased spontaneously, or by the pressure of the sponge, or compress, which was tied over the wound, the artery should not be interfered with. In by far the majority of cases, if proper precautions be taken, there will be no recurrence of the hemorrhage. The patient should be kept perfectly quiet, free from all causes of excitement, at perfect rest; and to ensure that the limb shall not be moved, a bandage should be carefully applied from the extremity of the limb upward, and a long splint secured. The flannel bandage being the most elastic, is the best material for such methodical pressure and support. Elevation of the limb will add much to the efficacy of the preventive treatment.

The ligation of an artery, which is the only sure precaution against the return of hemorrhage, is not only a difficult operation, requiring much skill for its successful performance, but when necessary to control the bleeding from a recent wound, becomes a very dangerous one to the safety of the limb or life of the individual. In cases of disease, nature, always on the alert, has enlarged contiguous blood-vessels, which are ready to assume all the functions of the one requiring obliteration. In a wound in a healthy person no such preparation has been made; and in cutting off the main supply of blood through a limb it becomes a very serious question, often answered by the loss of the limb and even life, whether the circulation will be re-established in time to save the member from mortifying. When a ligature is placed upon the main artery of a limb for disease, previous developments in the collateral circulation have been made to such an extent, that the extremity may not even lose temperature after the ligation, and as there is no diminution of the nutrient supply there is no fear of mortification. If placed on a healthy vessel for an injury, the limb at once becomes pale and cold, requiring the application of artificial warmth and enveloping in flannels to support life in it until the circulation be re-established, when the limb becomes actually warmer than its colleague. The arterial supply is now disseminated in vessels much nearer to the surface than before, where its chief channel was deeply embedded in the tissues. The rapidity of this collateral development in the limb is well exhibited in primary and secondary amputations. When a thigh is amputated in a healthy portion, very seldom are there more than three or four ligatures required to stop all oozing and render the stump quite dry. If the amputation be necessary at the same point three or four days after an injury to the main vessel has been received, the number is greatly increased: as many as twenty-eight arteries have been ligated by Langenbeck after amputating a thigh under similar circumstances.

Should active hemorrhage continue and show no disposition to cease, the wound should be dilated, the bleeding mouths of the artery found, and *a ligature applied both above and below the injury.* This has become the fixed practice and the only safe one, taking its place among the aphorisms of surgery. The universal adoption of this practice is not only based upon experience and observation, but could be determined *à priori* from the physiology and anatomical distribution of arteries.

All surgeons are familiar with the anastomosis or collateral circulation in blood-vessels. When the current of blood is stopped at any one point, it will soon find its way through many circuitous routes round to the very point through which its straight course had been checked. When an artery is divided, it is well known that, owing to its muscular and elastic structure, that portion above the wound at once contracts and retracts, so that the tube which was before cylindrical, now resembles a claret bottle with a much constricted neck. A clot of blood soon forms in this mouth and neck, and the passage of the blood is intercepted. In the lower portion of the divided vessel similar changes are going on, but not to so great an extent. The contraction (owing to the severing of the nerves which give tone to the arterial walls) is only partial, the walls being to a certain extent paralyzed, and so little blood remains in the tube that a very small and indifferent clot is formed. When the upper portion of the artery is firmly closed, preventing all egress to blood, the lower portion remains patulous, inviting discharge. As soon as the blood-currents find their way by circuitous channels, it wells up from the wound in a continuous purplish stream, all impulse having been lost, and also most of the oxygen by the long roundabout way which the blood now takes. The darkness of the blood will depend upon the difficulties of the circuitous passage; the rule, however, is scarlet or arterial blood from the upper end of the vessel, dark or veinous colored blood for its lower end.

Guthrie lays down the two following rules as the great principles of surgery, to be observed in the cases of wounded arteries, and which ought never to be absent from the mind of the surgeon:

1. *That no operation ought to be performed upon a wounded artery unless it bleeds.*

2. *That no operation is to be done for a wounded artery in the first instance, but at the spot injured, unless such operation not only appears to be but is impracticable.*

When it is necessary to ligate an artery, the surgeon must be guided by his anatomical knowledge, and by the pulsation in finding it. In dilating the wound so as to expose the bleeding mouths, the incisions should be made parallel to the course of the vessel, and sufficiently free to facilitate the search. The dissection is carefully conducted, dividing layer by layer, and avoiding the nerves and veins which always accompany the large arteries. When the bleeding mouth is so exposed that the origin of the jet of blood is seen, the vessel is transfixed by a tenaculum drawn out and secured as it would be in a stump after amputation.

Where it is impossible to ligate the bleeding vessel at the point wounded, a point should be selected, at which the vessel is comparatively isolated, easily discovered, and free from large collateral branches. *In exposing it make a free incision.* The common mistake that most surgeons make is a small incision, which hampers the search. When we approach the artery, use the grooved director to isolate those cellular layers in which the vessel is always found. The point of the knife should *never* be used for this purpose. The lips of the wound should be drawn asunder by an assistant, so as to give to the operator the light necessary for accomplishing speedily and successfully the ligation. In all cases requiring such an operation, it is desirable to have the patient completely under control, and, therefore, chloroform should be administered.

When the artery is found, and the ligature passed under it, before tying it be quite sure that it is the vessel, and it alone, and not the nerve that has been seized. To be satisfied on this point, it is only necessary to draw slightly upon the thread, and examine above and below to see whether the pulsation has altogether ceased below the ligature. Having determined that the thread is properly placed, it is then firmly tied, the ends are brought out of the wound and secured under a strip of adhesive plaster, attached to the immediate neighborhood of the wound. This mode of disposing of it will protect it from becoming entangled in the ordinary dressing, and be drawn upon when these are daily removed. Water dressings would be the proper after-treatment. The thread will have come away spontaneously, by the eighth, twelfth or sixteenth day, according to the size of the vessel ligated.

When it is necessary to ligate the artery in its course above the seat of hemorrhage, I would prefer using a fine silver wire ligature. This is well twisted upon the artery, and then cut off, leaving only the loop with one or two twists in the wound. The advantage is, that the foreign body being very small, not weighing more than one-third or one-half of a grain, creates but little irritation, and the wound can be healed in a few days by quick union. This will protect the patient from the dangers of suppuration, pyæmia, or secondary hemorrhage from the ligated point.

In the treatment of reducible inguinal hernia, where I have obtained permanent cures by sewing the columns of the ring together by silver wire sutures passed subcutaneously, the small loop of wire remains permanently in the inguinal region under the skin, and gives no trouble. From experience, in limited periods, I have reason to believe that it will remain innocuous for a lifetime.

The silver wire should not be applied to arteries in a suppurating wound, or where suppuration and sloughing must ensue, as in cleansing the wound it would be liable to be disturbed, and may be the cause of bleeding. Should the ligation of the large arteries at the root of the neck ever prove successful, it must be by the adoption of the silver wire ligature, which can be twisted sufficiently to cause a certain degree of irritation in the outer coats of the artery, and induce a copious deposit of lymph for incarcerating the wire and thicken these coats, without causing sloughing of the inner coats or opening the vessel.

Local treatment of wounds.—Having removed all foreign bodies, and hemorrhage having ceased, the dressing now required should be of the simplest description. It is known that gunshot wounds, favoring the contused variety, show a constant disposition to suppurate and often to slough. *This process of suppuration is not necessary to the healing of the wound, and should be kept in subjection as much as possible.* This is effected by the continued application of cold, which, by keeping down excessive reaction, and keeping out an excess of blood, diminishes the source of the pus supply, and thus hastens the cure. In former times, suppuration was considered essential in the healing of all wounds, by permitting the escape of so much poisonous matter, which had accumulated in the system, and which must either now find a vent, or, if retained, would be considered the satisfactory cause of any sickness which the wounded man may ever suffer from hereafter. The wound was therefore plugged with a lint tent, piles of greasy lint in cushions were applied, and after covering with a sufficient number of compresses and bandages, a forcing bed was formed, which supplied pus to the satisfaction of all interested; and it was common enough to see life drain away from this opening.

This smothering of wounds and smearing on of greasy ointments, which the wounded formerly encountered, was a second enemy, far more fatal than the enemy on the battle field; as in its ranks ranged exhausting suppuration, with its hectic; pyæmia, with its rapid poisoning; hospital gangrene, with its sudden collapse, and erysipelas, with its thousands of victims, broken-down constitutions, tedious convalescence, very protracted cures, and endless pain and annoyance.

How much more rational is the present practice. *Keep away all hot dressings, which invite blood to the part.* Vote poultices a curse, and eject the dirty, troublesome application. Guthrie says poultices should not be permitted in a military hospital; they are generally cloaks for negligence, and sure precursors of amputation in all serious injuries. With more recent writers they even meet with less favor.

The only dressing required for wounds, of whatever character, is the water dressing, and it should be used as follows: apply a single thickness of wet linen or cotton cloth over the wound, allowing it to extend over a considerable surface. If possible, cover this with a layer of oiled silk, waxed cloth, or india-rubber tissue. A second layer of cloth or a band secures the two former layers in position, so that they will not be displaced by the motions of the patient in sleeping. Then, either squeeze cold water frequently upon this outer cloth, which will keep up the low temperature; or what is a much more convenient and less laborious plan, suspend a bucket or some vessel containing water in the neighborhood of the wound, having a narrow slip of cloth, or, what is better, a lamp wick from the suspended vessel to the bandage upon the wounded limb. By capillary attraction, a constant stream of water is carried from the vessel to the dressing, and by its evaporation; robbing the skin of its animal temperature to get a sufficient quantity of heat to convert the water into aqueous vapor, it refrigerates the limb. The advantage of using the oiled silk, waxed cloth, or india-rubber tissue is, that should the water supply accidentally give out in the suspended vessel, the piece of cloth beneath it remains moist upon the wound. The wet cloth absorbs the discharges, and should be changed two or three times a day, it being well understood that they be disturbed as seldom as possible, compatible with cleanliness.

The surgeon should never be in haste to change the cold for warm applications. Should the virtues of a poultice be called into requisition, a soft wet compress covered with oiled silk and secured by a flannel roller or outer compress, is always at hand, and will be found to combine, in a simple form, all the properties of a poultice. It is light, moist, soft, and is kept warm by absorbing animal heat, which the oiled silk and outer compress retains. If we add to these, cleanliness, facility of medication, and the readiness with which an impromptu dressing can be made, we find an array of advantages which excludes all substitutes.

A more effectual mode of keeping down reaction is, by using ice bladders, which are placed upon the india-rubber, waxed or oiled silk covering. These are of very general application, and make the least call upon the personal attention of nurses. *Whenever ice is used, never apply it directly to the skin, but always through the intervention of compresses*, which may be made sufficiently thick to accommodate the application to the sensitiveness of the patient. When possible, these bladders should be of india-rubber or gutta-percha. A large supply of these should always be on hand. The animal bladder is a miserable substitute, as it is not only a very dirty application, allowing the water to ooze out and keep the patient constantly wet, but the bladders become very offensive, and are soon destroyed.

Cold water is the only proper and universal antiphlogistic that can be applied to wounds. It has the convenience of always being at hand, it keeps up a uniform action, is clean, simple, cheap, agreeable to the feelings of the patient, easily obtained, easily applied, demands least care from the nurses, who have their hands usually full, and is withal effectual. With the judicious application of cold the surgeon can defy inflammation. Cold acts by keeping down temperature, constringing vessels, and keeping blood from the part injured; so that inflammation, which consists in the engorgement of blood-vessels and an excessive supply of blood, cannot get a foothold. Heat, redness, pain and swelling, all depend upon congestion; control the supply of blood to a part, and inflammation is kept in abeyance.

As the advantages of cold water dressings are obtained through the evaporating properties of water, this action may be increased by medicating it with saline substances or alcoholic tinctures. Sugar of lead, sulphate of zinc, tannin, muriate of ammonia or laudanum, spirits of camphor, and, especially, tincture of arnica would be useful adjuvants. Whilst the irrigation is going on, the compresses next the skin may be moistened every three or four hours with any of the above preparations. Should the wounded patient feel chilly, the cold dressings will not be used until reaction has taken place. There are a few persons with whom cold water is not admissible. In all cases the feelings of the patient will be our guide as to the applicability of the remedy. When not grateful and refreshing to the patient, but, on the contrary, the cause of complaints, the irrigation must be superseded by a wet compress, covered with oiled silk or a waxed cloth. This will soon attain the temperature of the body, and will keep the parts moist and soft. The dressing requires to be changed twice in twenty-four hours; not that the compress would get dry, for the perspiration from the part which is kept in by the oiled silk would bathe it in a continual and permanent moisture. The object in changing is to get rid of this secretion, which, by decomposing, would irritate the wound.

A question of great moment is, when should we desist from water applications and change for some more useful or appropriate dressing? According to the present rational views of surgeons, no other dressing is ever required, however serious a wound may be. As long as inflammation threatens, so long is it necessary to prevent engorgements. As long as suppuration is kept up, so long will the efficacy of cold be required to constringe the blood-vessels and control the source of the purulent supply.

Pus, which we call a healthy fluid, is a heavy drain upon the system. It is made from the richest ingredients of the blood, which were intended for the repair of tissues. Once converted into pus, it is unfit for any further useful purpose, and is therefore a waste of precious material. This discharge is not more necessary to the healing of wounds than to the nutrition of the body. Extensive wounds, healing by the first intention, do very well without its intervention. Large subcutaneous wounds, when even their sides are not kept in apposition, heal with rapidity without the formation of pus. Under a scab we find tissues form, by what has been called the remodeling process, without it; and it should be our constant effort to heal all wounds, and I would say especially gunshot wounds, with the least possible discharge. Hence the water dressing can be continued beneficially for weeks, or as long as the wound remains unhealed. The most recent writers on gunshot wounds state that the wet cloth should be kept on until cicatrization is completed; and that no other application so protects and promotes the formation of new skin. There are a long list of ointments which have heretofore held universal sway in the treatment of wounds. All of these can be dispensed with for the more simple dressing. Should the wound require stimulation, the nitrate of silver wash, grs. xx to the ounce, when brushed over the part, will suffice; or tincture of iodine, or iron, or some stimulating astringent might be equally applied in addition to the water dressing, so that any imaginary condition of the wound might be successfully met by the medicated wet cloth.

The disturbing influences in the healing process of wounds are numerous, and most of them are capable of correction without much trouble. Among these are found imperfect transportation over rough roads in improper vehicles; bad attendance, such as rough or too frequent examinations; useless bandaging, which promotes infiltration; too frequent dressing; improper food; scorbutic, syphilitic, and other diseases; the moral depression of defeat, and above all, the imperfect ventilation and undue regard to cleanliness in the wards of military hospitals.

We have already said that a surgeon is never warranted in cutting down upon an artery and tying it upon suspicion—he must be an eye-witness of the hemorrhage, and see that it cannot be controlled by other means. The ligation of an artery is always a troublesome operation, and from the fear of subsequent mortification, always jeopards the limb, and necessarily with it the life of the patient. This is specially the case in recent wounds, before nature has prepared a collateral circulation, so that the rule which we have laid down is imperative, *never ligate an artery, however large, in which hemorrhage has spontaneously ceased*; and, moreover, that a good compress is usually sufficient, when applied immediately after the receipt of injury on the battle field, to stop the bleeding even from the largest vessels, when position, quiet, rest, and other prophylactics will prevent its return.

In the ordinary course of gunshot wounds, suppuration is established about the fifth or sixth day, when the track of the wound commences to be organically cleansed of all those tissues which have been crushed and so much injured as to be no longer preserved among the living tissues. During the elimination of these destroyed parts, where the precaution of rest and absolute quiet has not been enforced, hemorrhage, called secondary, appears. All injuries to large arteries threaten, sooner or later, to produce secondary hemorrhage. However large the artery reopened by this process, the escape of blood seldom occurs with an impulse, but flows away in a continuous stream, which marks its escape from the *lower* end of the vessel.

When hemorrhage, even from the femoral artery, has been arrested for twelve hours, the efforts of nature are usually sufficient to prevent its return from the upper portion of the artery, although not from the lower end of the vessel; so that when the main vessel of a limb is divided by a ball, once primary hemorrhage is controlled, the great fear is then from bleeding through the lower end of the artery, and from mortification of the extremity. Any hemorrhage, after twenty-four hours, would be considered secondary, and would require special treatment. As long as the wound remains open hemorrhage may make its appearance, and it is not until a cure is effected and the parts are cicatrized, that the patient is positively safe from this dangerous complication. Cases are recorded where it has occurred ninety days after the vessel had received injury. Unless the causes of this hemorrhage be perfectly understood, the rules laid down for treatment will not be duly appreciated.

In speaking of the behavior of the two ends of a divided artery, we have already stated that the upper end contracts vigorously, diminishes its calibre at the mouth, and for some distance up the tube, until it simulates in its proportions the neck and body of a claret bottle. The blood, impeded in its outward course, allows a clot to form, which, acting as a stopper, shuts up the open mouth. The plug is continued in the contracted artery to the first collateral branch as a clot of blood, which nearly fills its cylinder. The lower portion of the vessel, having been in a measure paralyzed by the division of its coats, which had cut off its supply of nerves, acts with much less energy. The diminution of its calibre depends more upon the removal of distension from its elastic walls than from the contraction of its muscular fibres. The result is, that it remains more or less patulous; and as the supply of blood from above is cut off, there is but little arterial blood in it to clot and plug it up. As soon as this barrier or clot is placed upon the main thoroughfare, at the upper wound, preventing the blood from following its accustomed channel, nature is at once busy, opening and enlarging the circuitous by-ways and alleys of the circulation, so as to restore the supply to the extremity threatened with starvation, or, in surgical parlance, mortification. As when upon a high road a bridge spanning a stream is destroyed, travellers seek a ford higher up by which they may return to the thoroughfare beyond the impediment, so the blood taking the nearest by-roads above, soon gets around the obstacle, and empties itself into the main channel below it. The blood here changed in its direction, and not opposed by valves, passes up as well as down the limb, and finding an open gate at the lower torn mouth of the vessel, escapes. This fluid, moreover, in its roundabout course, has lost much of its vivifying properties; much of its oxygen is gone, and carbonic acid, ammoniacal gases and the like, have taken its place, marred its brilliant color, and diminished its clotting properties. No material then exists for stopping up the vessel, as in the upper end of the divided artery, and the result is, that secondary hemorrhage nearly always occurs from the lower ends.

This being well understood, we can now explain why a ligature placed on the upper orifice alone, or on the course of the artery above the injury, should not stop but only temporarily control the hemorrhage. As soon as the collateral circulation above the ligated point is re-established, the lower opening in the vessel remaining as before, hemorrhage must recur, or, if this circulation is not re-established mortification must follow. *The rule then is imperative, ligate both ends of the vessel at the point wounded; this is the only safe course to pursue.* Another strong reason why the ligature should be applied to the wounded ends of the artery is, that there is always some uncertainty as to the vessel injured. The very serious and often fatal operation of ligating the femoral artery has been performed for injury to one of its branches, which had not been suspected until a post-mortem examination revealed the source of bleeding. When the ligature is applied to the bleeding mouths, this accident cannot happen.

The course which should be adopted in the case of an injured artery bleeding, is as follows: After the hemorrhage has once been controlled, through either some carelessness on the part of the surgeon or restlessness on the part of the patient, getting up to help himself when he had strict orders to the contrary, etc., or perhaps from rough transportation over bad roads, or the sloughing of the wound, hemorrhage reappears, the limb should be at once bandaged from the extremity upward, making careful, regular pressure, so as to diminish the quantity of circulating fluid. Over the course of the main artery, and for some little distance below the wound, a compress saturated or not with some of the styptic preparations of iron should be firmly secured, the bandaging of the limb extending to one or two inches above the injury. The patient is then to be placed upon his back, the limb elevated and an ice bladder applied over the wound. Absolute quiet should be enjoined, and secured by a large dose of opium.

In many cases, this dressing will bring about the desired object, when assisted by those internal remedies which control the force of the circulation, as veratrum viride, digitalis, etc. By the use of the compress saturated with per chloride of iron, in connection with absolute rest, I have succeeded in checking secondary hemorrhage from the carotid artery after the escape of the ligature. But should the parts be so situated that this pressure cannot be applied for a sufficiently long time, or should it not control the bleeding, then the proper course is to ligate the mouths of the artery in the wound without further delay. No case of secondary hemorrhage should destroy life by repeated recurrence; a surgeon is very culpable who permits life to ebb away from his grasp. Physicians cannot be too guarded against the delusive attempts at stopping the bleeding after the recurrence of secondary hemorrhage, it is certain to return and certain to destroy life, as experience repeatedly proves. Every fresh hemorrhage increases the dangers and doubles the risks, *therefore, never neglect ligating after the second hemorrhage.*

You must not be deterred from placing a ligature on the open mouths of an artery in a suppurating wound, on the deeply grounded, but erroneous idea, that the artery has had its coats softened by this process. Practical surgery shows conclusively, that the coats are tough enough to sustain a ligature in a suppurating wound, and therefore the rule should have no exception. *Ligate in the wound under any circumstances, when it is possible.* The swelling and infiltration of tissues, renders the search after the injured artery difficult, but the surgeon, who, looking to the side of humanity, considers it a sacred duty to do everything for the interest of the wounded, must not allow difficulties to interfere with his proper course. Safety lies alone in this operation. The difficulties must be met and overcome.

The following appearances will be observed in the wound, and will assist in the search : After dividing the infiltrated tissues, should the injury have been received over forty-eight hours, particularly if five or six days have intervened, the ends of the vessel will be found incarcerated in a mass of greenish yellow fibrine which indicates in a remarkable manner their situation. That which conceals the lower mouth of the vessel is always in smaller quantity. Where post-mortem examinations are made, a probe introduced into the artery from below would make its appearance at a point under the yellow patch, raising a thin portion as it protrudes; and should the patient have been destroyed by secondary hemorrhage, an opening will usually be found in this pellicle. Through the upper portion of the artery the probe would pass down with much more difficulty, owing to a contracted tube plugged with coagulæ—conditions which do not exist in the lower portion. These lymphy, yellowish green spots are, then, our guides after the wound has been freely dilated.

In a surgical operation, especially in ligating arteries, never cramp oneself from the fear of making too large an opening; the error is always on the other side. Having found and ligated the orifices, the water dressing should be continued as before, care being taken not to apply it should the limb become cool and pale. This is not usually the case after secondary hemorrhage, for the return of the bleeding indicates a re-established circulation, which the ligature at the bleeding mouths cannot now influence to the injury of the limb. Should it be impossible to find the bleeding mouths, after a long and careful search, then we will be reluctantly compelled to adopt the less satisfactory operation of ligating the artery above the wound; hoping that it may obviate further operation. Often, however, when this last plan has been adopted, a return of the hemorrhage necessitates a second ligature upon some higher point; and should this fail, as is not frequently the case, amputation of the limb will be the only resort to save life. Amputation must be equally resorted to if, after the application of a ligature, the circulation not being re-established, mortification of the limb ensues. In either case amputate above the seat of the ligature, so as to ensure a supply of blood to the stump for its nutrition.

These are some of the dangers incurred when the surgeon does not adopt the only proper course to stop the trouble at its commencement. Military hospital statistics show heavy mortuary lists where this rule is not recognized and followed. As the ligature acts as a foreign body, and must come away, it is of little importance what is used for that purpose, a strong cotton, flax or silk thread, fulfils all the indications required. When applied, it should not be interfered with until it has either come away of its own accord, or ten to fifteen days have elapsed, when cautious tractions might be attempted to hasten its removal.

Silver wire has been spoken of as ligatures for arteries. However well it may answer in fresh wounds where union by the first intention can be obtained, it is quite out of place in suppurating wounds, as when ligatures are applied for controlling secondary hemorrhage.

Punctured wounds made by the bayonet or sabre, require similar treatment. If the history and appearances clearly indicate the character of the wound, there will be no need of probing for imaginary foreign bodies. Such wounds usually bleed more freely than in gunshot. The hemorrhage is susceptible of control by the same means; pressure being preferred to ligation of arteries. The treatment should be cold water dressings, — irrigation preferred. Protect the wound from air if possible, by covering it with adhesive plaster, or collodion, and *dress it as seldom as possible. Once* probing of such a wound should satisfy the curiosity of any surgeon. A frequent repetition of this meddlesome surgery must end in mischief, beside the needless pain inflicted upon the wounded man.

Should a bayonet or sabre wound transfix one of the natural cavities, the internal injury may be rapidly fatal from hemorrhage, or the injury inflicted upon the contained organs may, sooner or later, lead to the destruction of the wounded by visceral inflammation. Under ordinary conditions, when such wounds exist in the extremities, where no large vessels are implicated, they require no special treatment. It is a class of wounds not as frequently met with in military surgery as one would suppose. The newly introduced sabre bayonet, when plunged into the body leaves but little work for the surgeon. Such cases seldom leave the battle field alive.

When the ordinary bayonet has buried itself deeply in a limb, suppuration may appear in the march of the wound. Should pus be suspected, and fears exist that it may be pent up under a fascia, it would be necessary to dilate the wound to permit of its free escape. Under no other condition, except for serious hemorrhage, where it is necessary to ligate the open mouths of the bleeding vessel, should a punctured wound made by either sword or bayonet be dilated.

Simple incised wounds, as sabre cuts, will be closed by adhesive plaster (or sutures which are preferable, should there be any tendency to gaping), to be followed by the cold water dressing. Should the wound be not of a serious character, it may be left even without after-dressing—the little oozing from its edges, when drawn together by straps or sutures, dries into a scab along the line of wound, and excludes air with its pernicious influences. This permits of the remodelling process, and cicatrization is effected without suppuration.

In gunshot wounds, the swelling which shows itself a few hours after the injury has been received, continues increasing until the completion of the third day, when it has attained its acmé with commencing suppuration. Should sloughing occur, it will show itself by the sixth or seventh. On the eighth or ninth day, the slough is in most cases separated from the edges of the track of the ball, and in a few days more will have disengaged itself. With the cleansing of the wound, the inflammation gradually subsides, the swelling diminishes, purulent discharge lessens in quantity, and the wound commences contracting. The middle portion of the track first closes, and with it, the opening of exit, leaving a funnel-shaped canal, which diminishes from day to day, becoming more superficial, until no depth is left to the orifice of entrance, which cicatrizes with a depression, marking distinctly the nature of the injury which has been received. This is the ordinary course which gunshot wounds take when judiciously treated in good constitutions.

The general treatment of such cases consists chiefly in interfering with the general health as little as possible. The commonly prescribed antiphlogistic remedies are, with but few exceptions, not required. The endless list of emetics, purgatives, diuretics, and diaphoretics, to which some European writers still cling with wonderful tenacity, can be dispensed with with benefit.

Guthrie, who represents this class, in speaking of the inflamed stage of gunshot wounds, says, that the treatment for subduing this should be active: "the patient, if robust, ought to be bled (if no endemic disease prevails), vomited, purged, kept in the recumbent position, and cold applied as long as it shall be found agreeable to his feelings; when that ceases to be the case, warm fomentations ought to be resorted to, but they are to be abandoned the instant the inflammation is subdued and suppuration well established."

Active purgation and vomiting are incompatible with that degree of quiet which is laid down as a fundamental rule in the treatment of gunshot wounds. As suppuration is usually long continued, and debility, with a certain degree of emaciation, usually accompanies the march of gunshot wounds, the disposition should rather be to harbor strength to support this drain than to despoil the system. The modern practice of support rather than depletion hastens convalescence, and is the only rational practice.

General and local blood letting are only required in a few special injuries of particular organs, which will be hereafter mentioned.

Emetics, as such, are never required in the general treatment of wounds. When very small doses of the emetic preparations are given, to induce relaxation and for generalizing the circulation, in this way deriving the excess of blood from the wound, they may be useful. Small doses of tartar emetic may, with other remedies, form a good prescription in cases of excessive reaction. Mild purgatives are in constant requisition, both for their detergent as well as derivatory effects.

The granulations of a wound are said to be a better index of the condition of the intestinal canal than the tongue, as they are much more impressible by any cause which induces an irritable condition of the system. Keeping watch over the digestive organs; preventing, by proper diet, any indigestible food from getting into them, whilst the excretions which empty into this great sewer are not allowed to remain and disturb the system, will be at all times judicious practice. Diaphoretics and diuretics are the milder antiphlogistic and derivative remedies, which may frequently be called upon to quiet the pulse and equalize the circulation.

The ordinary febrile reaction which so frequently follows the receipt of severe injury, should give the surgeon no annoyance *per se.* It is only a symptom, an indication of the extent of sympathy between the local irritation and the system at large. When, by judicious local treatment, the nervous excitement near the wound subsides, the pulse will, *pari passu,* lose its frequency and irritability. It is not a disease within itself, requiring to be especially attacked. In the general treatment of wounds, diet and rest are the two great remedies, which in by far the majority of wounds, even the most serious, are all that is required for successful treatment. Should there be an excess of general excitement, which a purge with a diaphoretic or diuretic is not able to quiet, we would administer to such, some one of that class of medicines which are known to control the excitement of the circulation, quiet the brain, and act as sedatives upon the nervous system generally, as opium, hyoscyamus, conium, belladonna, digitalis, veratrum viride, etc.

When local reaction is excessive, with great swelling and heat, there is a class of medicines which might be given with advantage. They act by increasing the tone of blood-vessels, and thereby cause a contraction in their walls and diminution of their calibre. Upon such remedies much reliance might be placed. Among these are found the mur. tinct. of iron, tinct. of belladonna, wine of ergot and others, which play a conspicuous part. It is by contracting the blood-vessels to such an extent that a sufficient supply of blood cannot be transmitted for the nourishment of distant tissues, that mortification follows the too liberal and long-continued use of ergot. By this property of producing contraction in blood-vessels, uterine hemorrhages are checked, or the action of the grand womb, with its immensely developed blood-vessels, excited. The entire profession have adopted the mur. tinct. of iron as nearly a specific, against the fearful inflammatory reaction of erysipelas; for stronger reasons, it is equally efficacious in simple inflammatory engorgements. Belladonna shows its general action by dilating the pupil—an effect explained by the change in the circulation of the blood-vessels of the iris. Its advantages in relieving injection of the blood-vessels of the eye are well known and largely used. It is spoken of as the remedy for the rapid relief of congestion of the spinal cord.

Although these are the individual effects of such remedies, they are not the specific action of these medicines. Their influence belongs to the economy, and in affecting all the tissues, those feel their influence most which are offending, as there would be the widest field for the remedy to show its common effects.

Inflammation is a perverted condition of the blood and blood-vessels of a part, which means a modified state of nutrition. There are two diametrically opposed means of correcting this condition and restoring health. One is, by reducing the amount of blood carried to the part which threatens to overwhelm the vital functions of such an inflamed portion of the body. This is effected by bloodletting, vomiting, purgation, abstemious diet, and the entire list of depletory or spoliative remedies, which weaken the enemy to such an extent as to allow of the part attacked successfully coping with the disease. But when the disease is conquered, the victory is as disastrous as a defeat, a long convalescence being required to restore the patient to his former state of health. The other method is, by increasing the tone, both of part and system, by supporting agents which strengthen the garrison, increase the vital powers residing within the tissues for resisting the encroachments of disease, and thus are enabled to drive out the enemy, however violently the attack may be made. These successes are attained with but little loss on the part of the system which comes out of the fire unscathed. Our object, then, should always be to cure disease by using such remedies as will cause the least possible loss to the economy.

In all injuries, were it not for an exquisitely sensitive nervous system, we would have but little systemic sympathy, and, therefore, but little personal annoyance. In the inferior animals, whose sensibilities are of a low description, limbs can be torn off without deleterious effect, and without producing inflammation. These inflammatory tendencies are only observed as we advance in the scale of animal life, until we find in man a perfection of a nervous system, with its corresponding susceptibilities to physiological as well as pathological impressions. If we could, by some metamorphosis in man, temporarily revert to the more primitive developments, we would diminish the dangers of local trouble; or if we could take possession, as it were, of the nervous functions and reduce them to their lowest stage for extending sympathies, we could equally keep down irritation, and to a great extent jugulate the tendency to establish congestion and, subsequently, inflammations.

Opium, by which we can effect this subjection, will ever be the greatest boon to the military surgeon;—it is a remedy which should never be absent from his reach. Going on the field, he should have his pockets well stored with it for immediate use; and in the entire treatment of the wounded it will ever hold a conspicuous place. Morphine is, perhaps, the best article for wounded men, as it has lost in preparation some of its astringent properties, which, as opium or laudanum, would produce too great a tendency to constipation.

The endermic method of using this remedy would prevent endless suffering on the battle field, or in hospital practice. When morphine is taken into the stomach, it is dissolved in the fluids there found, and then undergoes absorption. This takes place with greater or less rapidity, according to the nervous excitement under which the system is laboring. At times, its absorption is very slow, and its effects upon the system, from the small quantity found in the circulation, very indifferent. Under other circumstances, very large doses are administered in vain, to produce the soothing effects of the drug. It remains, perhaps, unchanged in the stomach; whilst under the same condition, if a much smaller dose, in solution, be injected under the skin of any portion of the body, its full effects are obtained in a few minutes. The following cases will show the marked efficacy of the remedy when used hypodermically:

Mrs. C. had been operated upon for cataract by division of the lens. Violent inflammation ensued, ending in the destruction of the eye, and for three days she suffered agony; day and night she was rolling about the bed in spite of repeated doses of morphine. Finding that one-half grain every two or three hours produced no alleviation of her suffering, I tried the experiment of injecting one-third of a grain under the skin covering the sternum. A Wood's endermic syringe was used; absorption was immediate; in two minutes she was relieved; in five, all pain had disappeared, and in ten minutes from the injection, she was sleeping soundly for the first time in seventy hours.

Mr. M. was accidentally shot in the neck with a Colt's pocket revolver. His head being turned, the ball entered the skin over the larynx, coursed downward and backward through the posterior triangle of the neck, and was found under the skin of the shoulder over the spine of the scapula, and removed. Considerable swelling and extravasation followed, which, diffusing itself, discolored that side of the neck. Some of the brachial plexus of nerves must have been injured, as the patient was soon seized with violent pains, shooting down toward the fingers, which, although never altogether absent, would increase to torture as evening advanced. Toward morning they would remit and allow of sleep, after a restless and painful night. Gum opium and morphine in large doses gave him no relief. The arm was so sensitive that he would not permit its being handled. One-fourth of a grain of morphine in three or four drops of water was injected under the skin of the shoulder; in five minutes all pain had left him, and his arm could be examined rudely without the slightest suffering.

By the use of this little instrument, a new and extensive field for doing good is open to the humane military surgeon, and he who is the fortunate possessor of this talisman, will receive daily the thanks and blessings of his suffering patients. When chloroform cannot be obtained, I would suggest this mode of blunting sensibility, immediately before operations are performed or painful and tedious dressings are made. It will be found a good substitute, and one which will yield its full effects without delay or trouble. There are very few injuries requiring operation which do not demand the free use of opium. Narcotising the patient immediately before the operation, and keeping him under its influence for some hours, is among the best means of preventing an excess of reaction. The rapidity of action when morphine is used endermically is a very great advantage on the field, where every moment is of value. For complete narcotism, where a sufficient quantity of morphine is used, five minutes are all that is required; whilst with chloroform we all know that, when under excitement, its inhalation is often extended from thirty to sixty minutes, and even longer—time which the field surgeon can ill spare.

CHAPTER VI.

Complications which arise during the treatment of gunshot wounds—ERYSIPELAS, *contagious and infectious character*—*Constant tendency to debility*—*Treatment, general and local*—PYÆMIA, *a rare disease in our country; symptoms*—*Theory of multipled abscesses*—*Great remedy; Prevention by rigid observance of hygienic regulations*—*Local and general treatment*—HOSPITAL GANGRENE, *its appearances, how recognized; causes giving rise to it*—*Thorough ventilation necessary to successful treatment*—*Local applications, actual cautery, etc.*—TETANUS *characters; march*—*Rarity of cure in military surgery*—*Local and general treatment upon which most reliance can be placed*—*Woorara in Tetanus*—HECTIC, *from long-continued suppuration*—PERMANENT AND PERIODIC PAINS.

ERYSIPELAS.—We have already entered, in detail, into the causes of secondary hemorrhage, which is one of the most alarming complications that can befal the wound. A second, that is to both surgeon and patient, is *erysipelas*. This disease appears to revel in the depressing influences which follows armies, and sometimes, as an epidemic, attacks all wounds, ravages limbs, and makes its heaps of victims. For several years, particularly during the winter months, erysipelas has appeared, at times, even as an epidemic in the States, especially in the middle region of country. Our troops can, therefore, hardly be expected to escape its ravages. Although it frequently occurs as an idiopathic disease, its most frequent exciting cause is a wound.

Gunshot wounds in patients debilitated by the many depressing influences of camp life, are peculiarly prone to attacks of erysipelas. The variety more frequently met with among troops is the phlegmonous, or as it is now called, the cellulo-cutaneous variety. It makes its appearance with violent inflammatory symptoms, intense swelling, tension, redness, pain, heat, and effusion. It extends rapidly from the wound as a centre, and soon covers a large area, accompanied by symptoms of inflammatory fever, with dirty, foul tongue, and deranged gastrio-intestinal secretion. It will be remarked that the pulse, although frequent and full, has no strength, and general prostration ensues at a very early day. Often by the fourth day the hardened œdematous tissue already feels boggy, indicating the extensive formation of pus and sloughs under the skin. The wound usually gives outlet to these at an early day. But as the disposition of the disease is not to localize itself, the active effusion thrown out in the extent of tissues undergoes a pusy conversion, which leaves this matter disseminated in all the tissues where the effusion had been poured out. It is in this manner that the extensive purulent dissection of limbs takes place; when the muscles are isolated, blood-vessels separated from the surrounding connections, bones exposed from their periostium, and joints opened, a general destruction of cellular tissue ensues. Shreds, or layers resembling strips of wet chamois leather may be pulled away. The extensive loss of support to the skin causes it to break down in sloughs, which makes a vent for the escape of this accumulating fluid. Nature, in its weakened condition, cannot stand this drain of its best nutrient material; and prostration, feeble, irregular pulse, dry tongue, diarrhœa, delirium, and finally coma, ends the scene. Or, should judicious treatment check its inroads, a tedious convalescence and a shattered constitution remains to the patient.

Erysipelas can always be recognized by its distinctive characters of widely extended local inflammation, with tendency to rapid suppuration and sloughing of the wound.

The prognosis of this complication is always serious, when it occurs after gunshot wounds, in military surgery, because the constitutions of the patients have been undermined, to a certain degree, by the hardships and irregularities which all soldiers in time of war must submit to.

In the treatment of gunshot wounds it must be remembered, that erysipelas, which is a very fatal complication, is often produced by a careless disregard of those hygienic regulations which are so essential in the proper organization of a hospital. Over-crowding, bad ventilation, want of cleanliness, are constant causes for its production and propagation. As the disease is clearly contagious as well as infectious, the directors of military hospitals must be very careful how they permit a case of erysipelas to be introduced into a ward with wounded men; for inoculation will at once ensue, and when erysipelas has taken possession of a ward, it is with great difficulty eradicated. Its effects can be traced first upon contiguous patients, whose wounds, healing kindly prior to the introduction of this focus of contamination, now take on erysipelas. The system soon shows the depression under which the patient is laboring. Some further complication, with low visceral inflammation of either the membranes of the brain or lungs or intestinal surface ensues, and life is overwhelmed by this combination.

Erichsen, in his Science and Art of Surgery, mentions the following case in proof of the contagion of erysipelas, as having occurred in one of his wards at University College Hospital. "The hospital had been free from any cases of this kind for a considerable time, when, on the 15th January, 1851, at about noon, a man was admitted under my care, with gangrenous erysipelas of the legs, and placed in the ward. On my visit two hours after his admission, I ordered him removed to a separate room, and directed the chlorides to be freely used in the ward from which he had been taken. Notwithstanding these precautions, however, two days after this, a patient, from whom a portion of necrosed ilium had been removed a few weeks previously, and who was lying in the adjoining bed to that in which the patient with the erysipelas had been temporarily placed, was seized with erysipelas, of which he speedily died. The disease then spread to almost every case in the ward, and proved fatal to several patients who had been recently operated upon." If such be its tendency in civil hospitals, how frightful will its march be among the wounded in military hospitals. Such cases should be kept exclusively to themselves, or they entail incalculable loss upon the wounded.

The antiphlogistic treatment of erysipelas, especially the phlegmonous variety which we are now considering, has for many years been abandoned; and he who attempts to cure erysipelas in military surgery by depressing agents, will pay heavily for his rashness. However violent its symptoms are, the surgeon must not be deceived. *It is a disease of marked debility:* its violent attack is only a mask to be thrown off in a few days, and often in a few hours. When the plan of attack is so well known, as it is in erysipelas, where a study of the natural history of the disease has invariably shown, in its march, certain and speedy prostration, the surgeon is highly culpable who does not commence with the earliest treatment to build up and support the system, and thus prepare it to withstand the depression which is so sure to ensue, and which, if overlooked, will be so fatal.

Prevention is always more judicious than cure, and, therefore, our first care should be—by the strict observance of those hygienic regulations for ventilation and cleanliness, and against over-crowding—to keep the wards of an hospital with so pure an atmosphere as to give no encouragement for this low class of diseases to intrude themselves. When a case appears, isolate it at once, and use every precaution against contagion. The sponges, bandages, etc., used by this patient, should be confined exclusively to himself; for if the same sponge be used for a dozen, they would all be as surely inoculated. Fresh air is indispensable in the successful treatment of this disease. Leave all the windows open for thorough ventilation, running the risk of catarrhal affections, which are trivial when compared to the serious character of the disease under discussion.

The treatment, ever having in view the steady, onward march of the disease to suppuration, sloughing, and prostration, unless a barrier is thrown across its path, should be from the commencement stimulating and supporting. This tonic course is prefaced by some mild cathartic to cleanse the bowels of impurities which rapidly accumulate in them, and excite healthy secretions from the digestive organs. For this purpose, the comp. colocynth pill would be a good prescription, although a dose of castor oil or sulph. magnesia, would, in the majority of cases, fill every indication. Without waiting the action of this cathartic, which is expected to have only a moderate effect, we at once prescribe what is now called the specific by many, and recognized as useful by all, the tincture of the muriate of iron, thirty minims, in a wineglass of water, every three hours. Besides acting as a general tonic, and also through its mineral acid upon the liver, promoting biliary secretion, it affects directly the blood-vessels, producing contraction in their walls, and a diminution of their calibre, relieving congestion, and preventing, to a great extent, effusions. I have seen it cut short a traumatic erysipelas of the face after an extensive operation for cheiloplasty, in thirty-six hours from its appearance.

In connection with the mur. tinc. of iron, and of equal importance with it, is brandy and nourishment. Erichsen says: "I have seen the best possible results follow the free administration of the brandy and egg mixture, to which I am in the habit of trusting in the majority of these cases." Its liberal use will restore strength, soften the tongue, and remove delirium. When the skin is dry and harsh, mild diaphoretics should be used, and as anodynes are always required in the treatment to allay pain and to give sleep, Dovers' powders would be a valuable agent. By adopting this course of attending to the secretions, keeping the bowels soluble, and supporting the system, even from the very commencement against that prostration which is certain, sooner or later, to show itself, this scourge in military hospitals will be most successfully controlled.

Considering the disease as one of marked debility, most reliance should be placed upon the general treatment. All local applications should tend to relieve engorgement. In the early inflammatory stage, before suppuration is established, painting the limb with the per chloride of iron, or a dilute tincture of iodine, or using compresses soaked with tincture of arnica, etc., would tend to promote healthy action. Cold water, by irrigation, or iced applications, would be as useful here as in any other engorgements. All of these applications may be accompanied with the methodically applied roller, which will compress the limb, and by its mechanical support prevent infiltration and congestion, and relieve tension and swelling. Sugar of lead lotions are highly lauded. Free incisions are recommended by many surgeons to relieve the engorged vessels. They give great relief to the patient, but it is a question whether they do not increase the irritation and hasten the suppurative stage, an effect not to be desired, as the entire armamentarium of the surgeon is directed against the formation of pus.

When pus has formed, which will be recognized by the doughy sensation of the parts into which the fingers sink when pressure is made, and a little later by fluctuation, incisions, sufficiently free to admit of the ready escape of pus, should be made, and stimulating water dressings continued to hasten the elimination of the sloughs, and diminish the amount of secretion. The tincture of arnica, or spirits of camphor, or Labarraque's chloride of soda, diluted with from six to ten parts of water, or diluted tincture of iodine, make an excellent stimulating application. Wherever pus shows a disposition to bag, it should be let out by incisions. As the skin, largely undermined, is disposed to slough extensively, it should be supported by properly applied bandages, which, by diminishing the cavity within, will prevent burrowing of pus, and cause the skin to adhere to the deeper parts as soon as adhesive action can be excited.

Pyæmia, a disease very common in Europe, and a scourge of their military hospitals, is a disease but little known among us, and therefore not likely to attack our wounded, unless we neglect necessary hygienic precautions. When it shows itself in a hospital, like its kindred disease erysipelas, it is not satisfied until it has swept off its hundreds, and is a pest hard to be got rid of. The great similarity in causes, symptoms and effects, are sufficient grounds for associating this with the large class of asthenic diseases, among which erysipelas and hospital gangrene are prominent. It is impossible to control the symptoms and prevent a fatal issue, when, as acute pyæmia, it seizes upon the wounded in military hospitals; it is therefore much more to be feared than its kindred disease just mentioned. Although this disease is always associated with wounds, no wound, however trivial, or however well advanced toward cicatrization, is safe from its attack until completely healed. The disease is supposed to be caused by the absorption of the ichorous fluids decomposing in the wound, which produces a general poisoning of the blood, rendering it unfit for sustaining the economy. It has been called an acute decomposition of the blood.

The phenomena which accompany this affection are, great depression of the powers of the system, and the formation of abscesses in various parts of the body. In the prodrome, which may precede the explosion of the disease by twenty-four or thirty-six hours, the patient is restless, anxious, ill at ease, with forebodings of impending trouble. He looks pale and sallow, has loss of appetite, and generally deranged secretions. The disease commences by severe chills, which, in the acute cases, are repeated with much irregularity. In the subacute variety, these chills appear at such regular intervals, followed by high fever and terminating in profuse sweats, as to induce the belief of malarial fever. In many cases the skin is hot, with a pungent feel, irrespective of the chills; in others, the chilly and feverish sensations alternate. The pulse is feeble; face pale, with anxiety of countenance and tendency to delirium; tongue foul, a tendency for sordes to collect on the teeth, and the tongue to become dry; stomach uneasy, with bilious vomiting, and thirst constant. The suspension of secretions gives a dull yellowish icteric tint to the skin. As the pulse becomes more and more enfeebled, the patient may complain of pains in his joints, simulating rheumatism, and simultaneous with these, a reddening of the skin, with swelling of the joints. Collections of a pusy character will soon after be detected, distending the synovial sacks.

Collections also occur in the cellular tissue, and even in the substance of organs. These form rapidly and without much inconvenience. Often, the swelling alone—which has appeared during the night, unaccompanied with pain, redness or heat—indicates that a large collection of pus has already taken place.

Whilst these symptoms progress, the wound usually becomes foul and sloughy, ceasing to secrete pus. This is not the invariable rule, as surgeons have noticed cases in which the appearance of the wound was no indication of the destructive disease which had laid its relentless hand upon the injured. The disease may even run its fatal course without material changes in the wound. Certain injuries are more likely to be followed by pyæmia, and those of bone are said to be peculiarly exposed. As in all such low diseases, typhoid symptoms ensue at an early day, and usually carry off the patient at the end of the first week. Often stupor comes on as early as the fourth day. An examination after death will reveal a rapidly advancing decomposition, with gas in the blood-vessels, and purulent collections in many organs, as the lungs, liver, spleen, kidneys, heart and brain. Similar collections are found in most of the large joints, beside the multiplied abscesses of the cellular tissue.

The theory of the metastatic character of the abscesses, or the sudden change of place of such deposits by absorption and redeposit has long been abandoned. Pus, we now know, to be a modified nutrient fluid, which, from an impairment of its vitalizing principle, falls short of its object of repairing tissués. This exudation leaves the blood-vessels under ordinary acute inflammation, and is drawn out by the excited tissues which are not able to consume the excess which they have demanded from the circulation. This fluid, now at rest without the blood-vessels, attempts a formation of its own, developing cells of this plasma, which simulate closely the white cells in the progressive development of the blood, and are supposed by some pathologists to be identical with them. This is pus. When the entire circulating fluid has become poisoned, its entire plasma or liquor sanguinis is impaired. It is from this plasma that the blood-cells are to be generated. The usual process of development is commenced, white cells form as colorless blood corpuscles, and when the continued development into the red or perfect cell is attempted, many failures occur. There are, besides, many which had exhausted their formative powers in attaining the degree of development necessary to perfect the white cell. These remaining as such continue in the circulation. When the blood of a pyæmic patient is examined, a very large number of such colorless cells are found in the blood, sufficient to modify its color, and it is in autopsies that the separation of these white cells from the generating fluid shows the deceptive appearance of pus in the blood, or emboli in the large vessels at the heart.

Blood in this condition, with an impaired liquor sanguinis, is unfit for its duties as a life-supporting fluid. The various tissues of the body, not receiving the kind of nourishment appropriate for their healthy function, become irritated. Nature tries to make up the deficiency in quality by quantity. The irritated parts are supplied with an excess of the impaired nutritive fluid, which, escaping from the capillaries, is received into the loose tissues. This is rapidly converted into pus, by the development of white or colorless cells in it, which is the height of vitality in such an exudate.

Experience, which sustains this view, shows the disease to be purely a blood poisoning; a general disease with its local manifestations, which are unimportant. When the blood has been thus thoroughly deteriorated, no remedy which art possesses can restore it to its former healthy condition, and the patient dies.

Our great remedy lies in prevention, the hygienic precautions of rigid cleanliness, thorough ventilation, good food, and proper shelter, without over-crowding, will, if properly insisted upon by the medical superintendent, go far to keep away if they do not altogether prevent the occurrence of pyæmia. Too much attention cannot be paid to the detail of cleanliness in the ward. The slop buckets, which are such a common nuisance, should be examined with care, frequently emptied, scoured daily with lime, and always kept covered, that the emanations arising from decomposing urine, which is very deleterious in hospital wards, cannot escape. The bed and body linen of the patients should be daily changed, doors and windows must be kept open. If any difficulty exists in this respect, from the inattention of nurses or fears of patients, it would be better to take out the sashes so as to ensure continued renewal of the atmosphere, day and night.

There is a popular dread of night air which should be exploded. The purest air we have in cities is the night air, and is the very article which is so much needed in hospitals. If the patient is properly covered in bed, there is no fear of his taking cold, or contracting other injury from the continued renewal of pure air. These precautions must not be commenced when pyæmia has already shown itself, but are those necessary to be taken wherever the seriously wounded are treated, or some low form of disease will soon break out. Any one who will visit, during the night, a ward filled with suppurating wounds, will perceive the degree of vitiated air, and see the necessity for free ventilation.

It is a bad principle to concentrate the seriously wounded; always scatter them over the building, mixing them in with inmates from other diseases. This increases the available space for the seriously wounded, and prevents the depressing effect of the concentrated emanations from so many extensively suppurating wounds. It is for a similar reason that we have already recommended that rooms should not be kept too long in use when occupied by the severely wounded. As the air becomes poisoned, the ward requires to be unoccupied two weeks of every two months, for cleansing and purification.

When pyæmia threatens to become general in a military hospital, the seriously wounded should be put, if possible, in tents, or be allowed double space in a constantly-ventilated room, and an additional quantity of nourishing food should be given out to the sick. Feeding the wounded on broths and other slops, is paving the way to the debility which is a precursor of pyæmia. All small operations should be avoided, and even the hasty opening of abscesses guarded against. The best protection against this disease is a whole skin. When the acute form of the disease shows itself, surgery can do but little to assist the patient. If it be possible, more benefit will be derived from changing the patient into fresh air than from any other remedy. Our entire reliance should be placed upon the stimulating tonics. Strong, nutritious, easily digested food, and opium to allay pain and restlessness, are the means required. The tendency to delirium should not prevent the free use of this last remedy, for although it would increase the difficulty if it be given in inflammation of the brain or meninges, it allays pain, removes restlessness, stops muttering, and induces quiet sleep, when given in cases of debility accompanied by delirium. As in erysipelas the acid preparations of iron, as a blood tonic, may be exhibited.

Although so little is to be expected in the acute form of blood poisoning, in the subacute or chronic pyæmia, much benefit will be derived from rigidly pursuing the course of treatment just marked out. By the stimulating and supporting plan, with change of air, many patients, after a long struggle, may be saved.

The important indication for local treatment in pyæmia is to prevent the accumulation of putrescent fluids in the wound by cleanliness—and the frequent application of chlorinate washes, which remove fœtor and stimulate the granulating surface. The abscesses which form during the march of the disease, should not be too hastily opened, as this course, pursued with the many collections, will induce rapid prostration.

Still another fatal complication to which gunshot wounds are liable, is *hospital gangrene*, the name being significant of the cause of this pest, as it is never seen as an isolated disease without the crowded wards of a hospital. It is highly probable that, like the former diseases which we have just considered, it is a blood poisoning, depending upon a foul, infected atmosphere, operating upon a depraved and enfeebled constitution. It seldom attacks the strong and robust, but most frequently those who have become debilitated by exposure, disease, want of proper food, intemperance, etc.; so that in a crowded hospital, when gangrene threatens to devastate the wards, you might select, in advance, the cases which will most probably be first attacked. Many surgeons consider it a constitutional disease, occurring from a strictly local cause, which is found within the walls of the hospital. All surgeons recognize its contagious as well as infectious character, and the facility of transmitting it by sponges or dressings used in common in a ward.

The facility with which the air of a ward or even hospital becomes impregnated with this poison, would show that animal exhalations, especially from those suffering under this disease, possess the power of diffusing it. Burgman reports, that hospital gangrene prevailed in one of the low wards at Leyden, whilst the ward or garret above it was free. The surgeon made an opening in the ceiling between the two, in order to ventilate the lower or affected ward, and in thirty hours three patients in the upper room, who lay next the opening, were attacked by the disease, which soon spread through the whole ward.

Guthrie, confirms the above by his experience, which, he says, left no doubt upon the mind of any one who had frequent opportunities of seeing the disease, that one case of hospital gangrene was capable of infecting not only every ulcer in the ward but in every ward near it, and ultimately throughout the hospital, however extensive it may be.

Both English and French surgeons, in the Crimean war, recognized the atmosphere as clearly the vehicle of its extension, and that its increase or diminution depended upon the crowded condition of the wards and the degree of ventilation. They, also, observed the certainty with which it increased when the same sponges were used for gangrenous and healthy wounds. It may be considered a thoroughly contagious disease.

Those who observe the march of the healing process of wounds, within and without hospitals, know how easily the one is cured, and with what difficulty a tedious cure is obtained in the other. Where the exhalations from many suppurating wounds are concentrated in a ward, the cicatrization of all wounds, even the most simple, are retarded, and contagion of any kind readily propagated.

In military hospitals, hospital gangrene will be recognized by the following appearances: Although the patient may have recently shown feverish symptoms, with loss of appetite, yellowish or pale skin, dirty tongue, and deranged bowels, the first appearance of the disease is recognized in the changes which the wound undergoes, which has led many to believe it to be, at first, a local disease, in time infecting the system. The granulating surface of a healthy sore, about taking on this sloughing phagedæna, becomes dry and painful. The florid hue of the granulations rapidly disappear, and is replaced by a dirty gray or ash-colored slough, which fills the wound and forms a pultaceous and adherent covering to the granulating surface. As this gray slough increases in extent and depth, the surrounding surface becomes œdematous, swollen and of a livid red or purplish color. This engorged appearance of the contiguous skin always precedes the advance of the gray slough. The edges of the ulcer are abruptly cut, undermined and everted, gradually assuming a circular outline, irrespective of the form of the wound prior to its invasion. The gray, tenacious mass, being formed of the mortified tissue, holds its place and cannot be wiped off, although it sways to and fro when any attempt is made to cleanse the wound.

The liquefaction of these mortified tissues soon commences, and a dirty, thick, highly offensive, irritating fluid, produced from the putrefaction of the slough, escapes from the wound, diffusing a peculiar odor which, when once smelt, will always be recognized. This is the poison which possesses such powers of infection when brought in contact with healthy wounds.

Once the disease has fairly rooted itself, its ravages are extensive and rapid. One can nearly see the extending line of slough, and often in twenty-four hours large portions of the skin, cellular tissue, and muscles will have mortified. These changes in the wound are accompanied by a severe burning, stinging, lancinating pain.

Pari passu with this local destruction the system is gradually or rapidly showing the influence of the poison. Although the symptoms may be at first of an inflammatory character, accompanied by a high fever, the pulse soon loses its strength, the mind is peevish, fretful and desponding, the tongue becomes dry and brown. The pain accompanying these changes is so severe as to deprive the patient of sleep. As the febrile accompaniments of the disease rapidly assumes a typhoid cast, delirium ensues and, with a tendency to coma, becomes a prominent symptom.

Should the case not terminate before the elimination of the sloughs commences, the separation of these may open large vessels, from which the hemorrhage will rapidly destroy life. The great nerves and arteries appear to resist the gangrenous destruction longer than the muscular or cutaneous structures. These yield in the end, and repeated hemorrhages close the scene.

I witnessed an epidemic of hospital gangrene, in Milan, during the summer of 1859. A large number of Austrian wounded had been put in a barrack prepared for their reception. They had undergone many hardships, retreating daily before a victorious enemy, and had, prior to the battle of Solferino, tasted no food for forty-eight hours. They had been deceived by their leaders, who had taught them that certain death awaited them should they fall into the hands of the Italians. With these impressions, the wounded hid themselves in the ditches and underbrush of the extended battle field, where many perished. Some were not discovered for two or three days, when they were sent to the hospitals. The previous hardships which the Austrians had undergone, their lymphatic tendencies, their irregular living, with the moral depression of repeated defeat, exposed them to the ravages of the lowest forms of disease. Hospital gangrene raged fearfully among them, destroying numbers. Many of their wounds were frightful from the extended sloughing, and their worn frames and gaunt visages indicated a fearful combat with disease. I was particularly struck with the mental depression under which many of them were suffering—amounting to despondency. This was further increased by the attendants and surgeons not speaking the German language, so that neither could their wants be known nor could sympathy be extended to them. From this combination of depressing causes, an epidemic of sloughing phagadœna appeared, which was appalling even to those accustomed to see disease in its most fearful form.

McLeod tells us that, in the Crimea, during the heat of the summer of 1855, not a few of those operated upon were lost by a gangrene of a most rapid and fatal form. All of those attacked by it were carried off. In the case of a few, who lived long enough for the full development of the disease, gangrene in its most marked features became established; but most of them expired previous to any sphacelus of the part, overwhelmed by the violent poison which seemed to pervade and destroy the whole economy. "The cases of all those who died in my wards seemed to be doing perfectly well up to sixteen hours, at the furthest, before death. During the night previous to death, the patient was restless, but did not complain of any particular uneasiness. At the morning visit, the expression seemed unaccountably anxious, and the pulse very slightly raised, the skin moist, and the tongue clean. By this time the stump felt, as the patient expressed it, heavy, like lead, and a burning, stinging pain had begun to shoot through it. On removing the dressing, the stump was found slightly swollen and hard, and the discharges thin and gleety, colored with blood, and having masses of matter, like gruel, occasionally mixed with it. A few hours afterward, the limb would be greatly swollen, the skin tense and white, and marked along its surface by prominent blue veins. The cut edges of the stump looked like pork. Acute pain was felt. The constitution by this time had begun to sympathize. A cold sweat covered the body, the stomach was irritable and the pulse weak and frequent. The respiration became short and hurried, giving evidence of the great oppression of which the patient so much complained. The heart's action gradually and surely got weaker till, from fourteen to sixteen hours from the first bad symptom, death relieved his sufferings."

In the treatment of hospital gangrene, we must consider it frequently a local disease, with rapid tendency to constitutional poisoning. One of our early duties would be to destroy the accumulating poisonous ichor in the wound to prevent further infection, whilst, at the same time, we correct those depressing causes which predisposed to the disease. Guthrie says, that constitutional treatment, and every kind of simple, mild, detergent applications, always failed unless accompanied by absolute separation, the utmost possible extent of ventilation and the greatest possible attention to cleanliness; and not even then without great loss of parts in many instances.

The local remedies act as caustics, and compose the most energetic of the pharmacopœia. The French and German military surgeons prefer the actual cautery to all other applications to check the encroachments of the disease, although Armand even speaks of this remedy, upon which much reliance was placed, as exceptionally checking the progress of mortification. "After a thorough cauterization, the eschar separates rapidly, and often exposes a second infected surface of greater extent." His individual experience gives the preference to tincture of iodine as a local application. The best results were obtained when a compress saturated with it was applied to the wound. Guthrie recommends the liberal use of the concentrated mineral acids, especially the fuming nitric acid. McLeod refers to the nitric acid as the most efficacious means of stopping the sloughing process. Laborraque's chloride of soda, pyroligneous acid, creasote, per chloride of iron, lemon juice, etc., are frequently used with benefit; but general experience in military surgery gives the preference to the mineral acid preparations. These are to be followed by irrigation, which washes away the ichorous discharges as rapidly as they form, and prevents further infection. Powdered charcoal, camphor and bark poultices are useful applications.

The local treatment alone, without the constitutional, would be followed by no good results. *The most important of all the constitutional remedies is change of air.* If the patient could be removed from the atmospheric influences of the infected ward, his chances for recovery would be greatly increased. Baudens states that without isolation all treatment will show itself powerless. Carrying the patient from the ward to a tent would be followed by immediate amelioration—fresh air being the great remedy. Keeping the intestinal action free by a little blue mass, or compound extract of colocynth, and the liberal use of tonics and stimulating diet, with wine or brandy and opium, will complete the treatment. Opium is required in every stage of the disease, and is administered in large and repeated doses to allay the pain, irritability and sleeplessness, which so generally attend the severe cases of gangrene. The diet throughout should be highly nutritious and should be liberally prescribed. McLeod, in his experience in the English service, states "that nitric acid, applied locally, and the exhibition of the tincture of the muriate of iron internally in half drachm doses, three times a day, proved to be the most efficacious means of stopping it, as it appeared in our hospitals."

It is thus seen that the three most fatal complications to gunshot wounds are the three kindred diseases, erysipelas, pyæmia, and hospital gangrene, all recognizing a common origin—viz., imperfect ventilation and want of proper attention to cleanliness, with the absence of those hygienic regulations necessary for the health of an army.

With proper care from the medical corps, these diseases, which are the chief scourges to the wounded, and the causes of nearly all the deaths, can be in a measure, if not altogether, prevented. Once they have made their appearance in a hospital, they will never leave until the building is closed, and the proper measures for purification resorted to. Prevention, in this instance as in all others, will be found better than attempts at cure, as many of these diseases, once they appear, are quite unmanageable, and tend naturally to a fatal issue. All of these diseases are benefited by the isolation of the patient in a pure atmosphere, when the infectious character of the disease is counteracted, and the patient is in the best condition for successful treatment. In all of them the antiphlogistic treatment cannot be too severely condemned. However useful such a course may be in a civil hospital, or in private practice, with patients unexposed to hardships, who are robust and have not been influenced by depressing agents, in a military hospital with the material which compose the inmates, an antiphlogistic course should not be thought of. The supporting plan, with stimulating tonics, is the only rational course that promises success, and should be used throughout the treatment. Attending to the secretions with mild remedies, allaying pain, and inducing refreshing sleep by means of opium, good diet, and due regard to hygienic regulations, will be the course of practice to be pursued.

TETANUS. — Another fatal complication of wounds, depending, however, upon very different circumstances from those recently considered, is *tetanus* or lockjaw: a disease fearfully malignant under any circumstances, and with scarcely an exception in military surgery. Fortunately, this is never an epidemic, nor can it infect a hospital, although pathologists have recently attempted to prove its origin traceable to an animal poison. This disease is much more frequent with us than it is in Europe, where it is rarely met with. In the Crimean service, McLeod mentions but thirteen cases as occurring in camp and in the hospitals.

This disease, which does not depend upon the size of the wound from which the patient is suffering, appears to be caused frequently by sudden atmospheric changes connected with dampness. Larrey, in his experience both in Germany and Egypt, found it in those wounded, who, after sustaining great exertions during the fight on a very hot day, were exposed to the cold, damp night air on the field, without shelter. After the battle of Bautzen, where the wounded were left on the field during the night, exposed to severe cold, Larrey found on the following morning that more than one hundred were affected by tetanus. In very hot climates it requires but little excitement to produce it—a trifling puncture or scratch is at times sufficient to cause an attack, and it has been noticed by military surgeons that the scraping of the skin by a ball, with bruising of the nerves, is more liable to this complication than the more severe wounds.

The proximate cause appears to be some injury to the nerves of the body, not necessarily connected with an open wound, as it has been known to follow the blow of a whip or a sprain. Wounds, in certain situations are thought to favor its appearance, viz., injury to the hands, feet, joints, etc. It may occur very speedily—a few hours after the injury has been received, or it may not occur for days. Rarely does it attack chronic wounds after the twentieth day. Its common period for appearing is between the fifth and fifteenth day,. when, perhaps, the simple wound has completely cicatrized. The premonition of uneasiness on the part of the patient, with vague fears of impending trouble, disturbed digestion, etc., are not often observed.

The first symptom which we usually recognize is a complaint of soreness of the throat, which, in ordinary cases precedes, by some hours, the contraction of the muscles of the jaw and pinching of the features. The spasm, instead of commencing in the injured part, always shows itself first in those muscles supplied by the fifth pair of nerves, and although in sudden and violent cases the spasmodic contraction of the muscles generally may rapidly follow the locking of the jaws, or appear to be even simultaneous with it, they are never found to precede it. The locking of the jaws; the contraction of the muscles of the neck, especially the sterno-cleido-mastoid, which, by bounding under the skin, accurately defines the triangles of the neck; the hardened condition of the abdominal muscles, the knots formed over the region of the recti muscles during the paroxysm; the stiffening of the muscles of the legs, whilst those of the arms remain free; the sardonic expression of the face; clear brain; sleeplessness; profuse sweating; incessant desire to drink, and difficulty in accomplishing it; with the occurrence of paroxysms of violent muscular contraction every few minutes, with loss of strength in the pulse, and rapid prostration, define the disease so accurately that it becomes one of those most easily recognized.

Any one who has ever felt a cramp of the calf muscles, may have a faint appreciation of the intense pain which a permanent and violent cramp of all the muscles must produce—a pain sufficient to destroy life promptly, through nervous exhaustion.

The prognosis of this disease is so serious, and the treatment, however conducted, so unsatisfactory, that many surgeons of large experience have never cured a case of traumatic tetanus. That fruitful source of information, pathology, gives us no instruction in this disease. An autopsy reveals nothing commensurate with the intensity of symptoms. A slight congestion of the spinal cord and medulla oblongata, is all that can be discerned. From the symptoms, we judge of the disease as one of intense nervous irritation. Recognizing the exhaustion which so soon shows itself, the treatment as laid down by the most recent authors, and the one now generally adopted, is one of support to both the nervous and muscular systems.

Larrey has cut short the disease in its incipient stage by amputating the limb, or dividing the nerve which is supposed to be at fault. Other surgeons, by isolating the irritation, have been equally successful. Such results are, however, rarities in practice, the operation often failing when performed at the very commencement of the symptoms, and always when the disease shows confirmed general spasms. At times, patients suffering from tetanus get well under the most varied treatment. Nearly every powerful remedy in the pharmacopiœa has been recommended as a sovereign cure by those who may have derived some benefit from such in the treatment of tetanus. Disappointment is sure to follow the confidence placed in any of these articles. The most judicious course is to disclaim all specific remedies, and be guided by the symptoms; allay, if possible, the intense nervous excitement, and support the system against the ensuing exhaustion.

The local treatment should consist in examining the wound for foreign bodies, and removing them, if possible, as they are frequently the exciting cause of nervous irritation, under the presumption that unless the local cause be removed we can expect but little abatement of the general tetanic excitement. Should no foreign body be found, if it be possible, an incision may be made on the cardiac side of the wound, to divide the nerves implicated, and paralyze their sensibility. The powerful acids and the actual cautery have been recommended for the similar purpose of destroying the excited nerves at the seat of injury. A solution of morphine, atropine or kindred preparations, may be instilled into the wound for their sedative action, and the simple water dressing continued.

The constitutional treatment will have for its object to remove all general and internal causes which may keep up excitement. *We should constantly bear in mind that tetanus is an affection of debility*, and that the violence of the spasmodic paroxysm gives a *false* appearance of strength to the patient, whilst the principal source of danger and death is from fatigue, induced by the energy of the muscular movements and the consequent want of rest.

As the bowels are always constipated and loaded with offensive fœcal collections, which might assist in sustaining the excitement of the nervous system, they should be at once emptied by a large dose of calomel, with gamboge, aloes, or scammony. When a difficulty is found in administering this, from the locked condition of the jaw, one or two drops of croton oil can be placed within the teeth, when, mingling with the saliva, it will be swallowed. Three or four times the ordinary dose will be required to relieve the torpid bowels. The patient should then be kept perfectly quiet—if possible by himself, as the stirring about of persons, noises, draughts, etc., excite sudden and repeated paroxysms of spasm. Ice bladders, blisters, or chloroform applications, may be made to the upper portion of the spine to allay, if possible, the irritation of this region.

Although opium is universally administered as

an internal sedative, its effects are not often obtained even when given in large doses. It is believed that it often remains unabsorbed in the stomach, and, therefore, without action. The same for conium hyoscyamus and the entire class of sedatives when given in the form of pill or extract. Unless medicines are given dissolved, they are not likely to be absorbed, or they are taken up so slowly that their good effects are not perceived.

Recently, in two cases of traumatic tetanus, I have tried the hypodermic administration of morphine in $\frac{1}{3}$ grain doses, dissolved in a few drops of water, and injected by means of a Wood's syringe. The effect of the remedy in a few minutes was decided, but was not persistent; partial relaxation of the jaws could always be effected, so that nourishment might be taken, and sleep could, also, be induced. It is by far the preferable mode of using opium, as its effects can be speedily and with certainty obtained. In one case, in which I injected 1-10th grain of atropine under the skin of the arm, the effect upon the pulse was so immediate that, in five minutes, it had increased from eighty to one hundred and fifty beats. It rapidly affected the salivary and mucous glands of the mouth — diminishing their secretions without, however, producing dilatation of the pupils or causing relaxation of the muscles. As no beneficial effect followed the atropine injection, morphine had to be used, when relaxation to a certain extent was immediately obtained.

The liberal use of belladonna has been recommended, and, from its great utility in relieving congestions of the lower portion of the spinal cord, we might naturally infer similar good effects for the medulla oblongata. The tincture of canabis indica has been highly extolled. Some cases have recovered under its use, but a very much larger number have died in spite of its administration. Stimulating and nourishing fluids must be liberally administered at regular intervals, and, notwithstanding the difficulty in swallowing, *the nurse should insist* upon its being taken. Many a fatal case can be laid to the charge of carelessness in nursing, where the wishes of the patient are permitted to regulate the nurse's duties. Beef tea, eggs, milk, custards, egg-nog and wine must be frequently poured down the throat of the unwilling patient, and, if the mouth cannot be sufficiently opened, the inhalation of chloroform, or the endermic use of morphine should be used to effect it. I have seen excellent results with either of these relaxing agents.

I have found porter an excellent tonic in such cases, as it combines both sedative, nourishing and stimulating or supporting properties. Under the frequent inhalation of chloroform, the spasms can often be kept under control.

By pursuing the above course of keeping the patient quiet, using sedatives with forced nourishment, and relieving the loaded intestines by croton oil, I have had the good fortune of saving three tetanic patients out of six cases which have come under my personal observation. As the three first cases which I treated were all restored to health, although they were very severe, I imagined that I had found a successful mode of treating tetanus, and published the same in the Charleston Medical Journal for 1857. Since that time, I have had three cases under observation and lost them all, notwithstanding the same course was pursued as in the successful cases.

When the patient is able, constant smoking of strong segars may be useful in quieting the excited nervous system. The impression among many observing surgeons is, that the patient is destroyed by exhaustion, called by some starvation. It is known, that if the patient can be kept alive to the sixth day after the attack, there is a likelihood of his recovery, and that by the tenth day he may even be considered convalescent. If the debilitating effects of the disease can be counteracted by the free administration of very nutritious food, such as brandy and eggs, etc., many surgeons believe that the nervous irritation will wear itself out. It is based upon this belief, and the known failures of the spoliative plan of treatment, that the above plan is now recommended.

Woorara poison has been recommended as an antidote from its known powerful sedative nervous action and its marked influence in counteracting the effects of strychnia. When poisonous doses of these substances are given conjointly, no poisonous effects are observed. The striking similarity between the spasms produced by strychnine and those of lockjaw, suggested the use of woorara in this latter disease. As experiments proved it efficacious in the tetanus of animals, its field of usefulness was enlarged to the human subject. Several cases of its successful use in chronic tetanus are reported. There is much difficulty in obtaining good specimens of this remedy. As no two possess similar properties, each must be tested by experiment before it can be tried upon the human subject. Cases are reported where its use hastened the death of the patient. It was first used by inoculation, now it is administered in the form of a mixture: ten grains of the woorara to a six ounce mixture—a tablespoonful every half hour until perfect relaxation is produced. Should poisonous effects, with death-like symptoms, show themselves from an over-dose, artificial respiration will support life and sustain the action of the heart until the poison is eliminated from the circulation by the kidneys. The rationale of the remedy is to keep the spasms from killing the patient by their violence, until the morbid state calling them into play has exhausted itself.

The not unfrequent sequela of severe gunshot wounds is long-continued discharge, producing emaciation and hectic, with its gradual dissolution of body and soul. It is not at all surprising that the daily discharge of a wound, when at all profuse, should cause debility, as we have already characterized pus as the nutritive essence of the circulating fluid. If the surgeon, who has many suppurating wounds under his care, overlooks the fact that he must make allowance for this drain and feed the wound as well as the patient, the wound being more imperious in its demands than the economy, deprives the latter of its due supply of nourishment, and progressive starvation must follow. It is on this account that what is called the antiphlogistic treatment, when fully carried out in the treatment of suppurating wounds, is injurious, and that the supporting plan is required. With diet, we have a powerful weapon for weal or woe in surgical practice. Soon after injuries have been received, when reaction runs high, by abstemiousness we can do much to quiet excessive irritability. But as soon as this stage has passed, and suppuration has become established, then the course of diet should be modified; now, liberal diet is necessary to prevent the febrile complication, which, in the early stage of the wound, abstemiousness controlled.

The use of an abundance of strong nutritious food, by enriching the blood, will increase the vital properties of the plasma, improve the tone of the tissues, stop the excessive demands of the irritated wounded parts, and diminish the drain. This treatment, with the liberal use of the astringent tonics, and the injection of stimulating astringents into the wound (as nitrate of silver, ten grains to one ounce of water, or tincture of iodine, or the acid tinctures of iron diluted, one part to five of water), will gradually diminish a discharge, which, under less supporting treatment, would continue for a much longer period. The economy cannot withstand this constant drain; it becomes irritable in its weakness. In its efforts to throw off the yoke, it still further enfeebles itself. Daily fevers, with their profuse sweats, reappear with fearful regularity. Finally, the blood becomes so poor, that it deteriorates rapidly, and the useless material which is ejected from the circulation, irritating the organs through which it passes, causes diarrhœa, and also copious deposits in the urine. The quadruple drain from wound, skin, bowels and kidneys, cannot long be resisted. Debility gradually increases, the patient rapidly wastes to a living skeleton, having literally melted away, and at last dies from sheer exhaustion—the conjoined result of mal-nutrition and wasting discharges. Such is hectic fever.

Another sequela of gunshot wounds is more or less *permanent or periodic pain* in the injured limb, connected or not with paralysis of certain muscles, the nervous supply to which has been impaired by the ball in its passage. When a nerve has been completely divided, permanent paralysis, with atrophy of the muscles, ensues—the limb gradually dwindling, if the muscles, indirectly destroyed, be important to the common movements of the extremity. A bruising of the nerves, without division, is also followed by a paralysis more or less persistent, which time, however, and stimulating embrocations will, to a great extent, remedy. This is not so much the case in sabre wounds. Where a nerve is divided by a sharp, cutting instrument, when the tissues are not displaced and the wound heals without suppuration, both experiments upon animals and experience in man show that a reunion of the ends of the nerves is effected, and nervous action restored to its former integrity.

When nerves are pricked, or in any other way injured without complete division, very severe neuralgic pains, with spasmodic action of the muscles of the limb, ensue. These pains extend up and down the injured limb, and, as in cases reported by Guthrie, have, with irregular intermissions, annoyed the patient for years. In one case, although the severity of the symptoms subsided after six or seven years, annoyance was, at times, experienced forty years after the injury had been received. A coldness of the parts supplied by the injured nerve is not an uncommon effect, and is more or less persistent. Sudden changes in the temperature, cold weather, or mental excitement, are among the exciting causes of such attacks The best means of mitigating the suffering, independently of the application of warm flannels, is the free use of stimulating narcotic embrocations. Any combination from the many articles of the materia medica, of stimulating and narcotic, or anæsthetic ingredients, would fulfil the indications of treatment. The internal use of quinine, aconite, hyoscyamus, belladonna or opium, will blunt sensibility.

The endermic use of morphine in one-fourth grain doses, or aconitine, one-sixteenth of a grain dissolved in two or three drops of water, will give immediate relief—in some instances a permanent cure has followed the first injection. Great reliance will hereafter be placed upon this new method of treatment. A complete division of the nerve at fault has been recommended, and practiced with some good results; but the divided nerve is liable to become diseased, or its cut ends swell into a neuroma, which, incorporating itself with the cicatricial tissue, would, from the amount of pressure exercised by the new formations, allow of only temporary relief.

CHAPTER VII.

Treatment of wounds of the different parts of the body, or topical surgery—Wounds of the head; Concussion; its characters and treatment—Compression; its symptoms—Variety of wounds of the head; their prognostic value—Simple wound of the scalp; treatments—Fracture without depression; course to be pursued when inflammation of the brain threatens—Fracture, with depression, to be treated without an operation—Trephining very rarely called for—Compound fracture, with depression and compression; trephining even here of doubtful propriety—Perforating wounds of the cranium complicated with foreign bodies.

Wounds of the head, when received in battle, require a special treatment, which cannot be engrossed in the routine practice for wounds. Owing to the proximity of the brain and membranes, and the facility with which shocks or direct injury can be transmitted through the protective envelopes, injuries of the head possess a peculiar significance. All wounds of the head are more or less serious, as the surgeon can never know in advance whether the brain be injured, and what amount of irritation or inflammation will ensue upon such an occurrence. Hence the necessity of caution in prognosis and treatment, which the experienced surgeon will always exhibit, however trivial the wound may appear.

Injuries of the head would divide themselves into those produced from shot, those from the bayonet or clubbed musket, and those caused by the blow of a sabre. Wounds are found of every grade of intensity, from a simple scratch to extensive destruction of the soft and hard parts, with or without those phenomena recognized as concussion and compression. As these terms will be continually referred to in speaking of the treatment of head injuries, we will, in brief define the meaning which the surgeon attaches to them.

Concussion, or stunning, appears to be a shock to the brain by which its substance is more or less shaken, with interference of its circulation, and often injury to its structure—its functions being suspended for a certain period. Immediately as an injury upon the head has been received, if at all severe, the patient is knocked senseless. He lies perfectly insensible, motionless, and all but pulseless. His face and surface becomes pale and cool; the breathing, although feeble, is regular and easily perceived; the pupils irregularly contracted or dilated; sphincters are relaxed, in common with the entire voluntary muscular system, so that the contents of the bladder and bowels often escape involuntarily. After continuing in this condition for a few minutes, hours or days, he gradually recovers consciousness. The heart first regains its accustomed action, the pulse gradually undergoes development, and the skin becomes warmer. At this period vomiting usually comes on, which arouses the action of the heart. This organ, under the excitement of emesis, drives blood to the brain, and with this free supply of stimulus to the general controlling organ, the patient rapidly rallies.

This is the common picture of concussion as seen in surgical practice, and the combination of its symptoms will be more familiarly recognized as those of ordinary fainting or syncope. The extremes would be those cases in which the patient staggers, but, after supporting himself for an instant against some house, fence or tree, recovers himself and, without further annoyance, continues his employment; or those in which the patient is picked up apparently dead, with relaxed muscles, pale surface, glassy eye, scarcely perceptible pulse and very feeble and irregular respiration. The death-like appearance becomes more and more confirmed, the breathing gradually ceases, and the pulse imperceptibly flitters away, without any sign of consciousness from the moment of injury.

In fatal cases, where concussion had been present, the brain has been found more or less injured, and so highly congested as to exhibit a dusky hue. Fissures have been found in its substance, or extravasations of blood in numerous or concentrated spots. In certain instances the brain has apparently shrunk from the excessive shaking or vibrations to which it has been subjected, so that it no longer fills the cavity of the skull. In some fatal cases where the brain had been fissured, the commotion among its particles had at once annihilated its functions, so that the heart's action had instantly ceased and no blood had been driven to the mangled brain to be extravasated into its substance. In cases of nearly instantaneous death from concussion or stunning, the brain, on examination, appeared in every respect healthy. On the other hand, in cases of perfect recovery after concussion, where the patient had lived some time (weeks or months) in the full enjoyment of all of his faculties, and had died from some disease totally foreign to the former head injury, extensive lesions have been found in the brain, and traces of large and extended extravasations of blood covering the hemispheres as well as in the cerebral substance. The irritable condition of the brain in which the patient is often left, after concussion of limited duration, with the impairment of memory, or of some one of the special senses or even partial paralysis, would be physiological proof of cerebral injury. Although its symptoms are usually transient, we may, doubtless, consider it a contusion or interstitial laceration of brain substance.

As this is an alarming condition, to those not familiar with the march of such lesions, those interested in the injured man are always clamorous for active interference, and it is with difficulty that the surgeon can free himself from the urgent solicitations of friends who believe that, unless prompt means are used, the accident must terminate fatally. The surgeon, under such circumstances, requires all of his presence of mind, and with firmness pursues strictly the non-interference plan of treatment. The course which rational surgery now recommends is to lay the patient horizontally, with his head perhaps a little lower than his body, so that the brain may have the benefit of gravitation to assist in its supply of blood. He is wrapped in warm blankets, hot bottles are placed around his body, and dry frictions may be used to excite the re-establishment of the circulation in the extremities; but beyond this the surgeon should not interfere. *The safest practice consists in doing as little as possible. The use of stimuli on the one hand or bleeding on the other are to be especially and studiously avoided.*

Only a few years since bleeding was the practice in stunning, and the amount of mischief done by this universal mania for bloodletting was often irreparable. We might as well bleed in a fainting fit and expect good results. We find, as in syncope, that the heart scarcely pulsates; so little blood is driven to the surface that it is pale and cold. The same for the brain where so little blood circulates that, from want of its proper stimulus, its functions are temporarily suspended. Were it possible to draw away much blood, the cessation of the nervous functions would become permanent. Modern surgery, in studying the natural history of disease and injuries, sees now, what it should long since have recognized, that nature, in her desire to harbor the circulating fluid, tries to put a safeguard against the rashness of surgeons, by shutting up the bulk of this living fluid in the inner recesses of the body, where it cannot be easily despoiled. On account of this change in practice, we now seldom hear of deaths from concussion, which was comparatively of common occurrence a few years back.

As regards stimulation, we must also desist as long as it is possible, and, when its administration is compulsory, give it with a most cautious, sparing hand. Remember that the degree and duration of shock depends upon the extent of injury which the brain has received, and that nature, always the most skilful physician, adopts this concussion as a safeguard to prevent further lesion. How are we to know that the brain has not sustained severe injury, extensive bruising or laceration, and that this extreme depression of the brain, with consecutive control of the heart's action, is not especially indicated to prevent hemorrhage within the brain substance and rapid death from compression by extravasated blood. We know this, that after severe injury to the brain, when, through officious meddling and the free use of brandy, the symptoms of concussion early disappear, violent reaction is induced, and internal hemorrhage or violent inflammation soon shows itself; and that, for the doubtful gratification of seeing the patient rapidly revive, we have the mortification of seeing him as rapidly destroyed.

Cases of concussion, absolutely requiring stimulants, are but very, very seldom met with in practice. Even when of a very severe form, all that is necessary, in the vast majority of cases, is to apply warmth to the surface, and carefully to watch the case.

Should it so happen—but this occurs very rarely—that the patient is manifestly in danger of sinking from depression of the circulation, then stimulants must be resorted to. As long as the pulse does not lose its strength under concussion of the brain, desist from active interference, should the insensibility last for hours or even days. After-trouble will be avoided by allowing nature to take its own course unmolested. When from the great and long-continued depression stimuli are called for to prevent threatening dissolution, their effects should be carefully watched, and as soon as reaction is apparent, with an im-improving pulse, at once desist from further interference. As is the state of depression, so will be the state of reaction. When the depression is extreme, the reaction will be correspondingly excessive, and, especially so, if stimuli have been freely administered.

When the patient has recovered from the state of insensibility, he should be kept perfectly quiet, excitement of every kind should be carefully avoided, the diet should be abstemious, the head kept cool, and tendency to constipation corrected; but, beyond this, no treatment is required until expressly called for by excessive reaction, with symptoms of congestion or inflammation of the brain. The precautionary bleeding, with repeated doses of calomel, to keep off symptoms, which, in the majority of cases, would not have occurred, was the routine practice of the old school, and cannot be too severely criticised. The complications which might arise in injuries of the head, after more or less serious concussion, will be hereafter considered.

Concussion is always simultaneous with the blow, and gradually decreases, if death does not carry off the patient early. *Compression*, the condition with which it is often allied, usually comes on some little time after the reception of injury, although it may appear either at the moment, or may not show itself for days or even weeks after the injury. The name explains the lesion. Compression is pressure made upon the brain, either by a portion of the skull or some foreign body driven into or upon the cerebral mass; or by an escape of blood from some torn vessel, which, by forcing itself into the unyielding skull, compresses its contents, or by effusion of lymph or pus, which inflammation causes to be deposited within the cavity of the skull. The symptoms by which this condition would be recognized, are as follows:—The patient lies in a state of coma, stupor, or lethargy, being paralyzed more or less completely, both as regards motion and sensation. He is heavy, insensible, and drowsy, at times answers mutteringly when rudely shaken or loudly spoken to, but immediately afterward is again breathing slowly, heavily and laboriously, as if in deep sleep. Should his face be examined, the lips and cheek on one side will be found to flap, during expiration, with a blowing sound, as if smoke was being blown from the mouth as in smoking. There is paralysis of that side of the body opposite to the seat of injury, and as a necessary consequence, both in expiration or in attempts at speaking, the corner of the mouth is drawn over to the sound side. The countenance is usually pale, cold, and ghastly, although it may be flushed with a hot and perspiring skin, the eyelids are partly or completely opened, with the pupils dilated and insensible to light; the pulse is slow, the heart acting under great oppression; there is constipation from torpidity of the bowels, with involuntary discharge of the fæces. From want of action in the bladder the urine is retained, and unless drawn off will decompose within the organ, when, from accumulation, either the bladder will rupture with poisonous infiltration, or the blood becomes poisoned from absorption. These symptoms are not always equally marked—the degree depending upon the cause. Unless the causes of compression be removed, the case usually terminates fatally, although cases are not rare, in which, after weeks of unconsciousness, reason has gradually been restored—the accompanying paralysis slowly disappearing.

Having now explained the two conditions of concussion and compression, which so commonly accompany severe wounds of the head, we are better prepared to study this special class of injuries.

The divisions which experience has proved of practical utility, are:

1. *Injury to the soft parts alone, uncomplicated with injury to skull or brain.*

2. *Wound of soft parts, with simple fracture of the skull.*

3. *Wound with depressed fracture of the skull, but without symptoms of compression.*

4. *Compound depressed fracture of the skull, with symptoms of compression of the brain.*

5. *Perforating wounds of the skull, complicated with foreign bodies.*

From the peculiar formation of the skull and the resistance which it offers to blows, unless a shot strikes it fairly at right angles, it does not perforate; but whether it be a grape, musket, or pistol ball, it flies off at a tangent, or, running beneath the skin upward, downward, or laterally, escapes. The head may even be struck with a round shot without serious injury. The patient may, or may not be knocked down by the blow; severe pain is felt, and a puffing up of the part instantly follows. When the hair is removed, although there may be no discoloration of the skin, there is abundant evidence of subcutaneous lesion, which, unless counteracted, will soon develop inflammation and extensive suppuration. The severity of the blow upon the head may have knocked the patient senseless: and in this condition, he is found by the litter carriers.

The transportation of head injuries requires great care, and the best transports should be devoted to this service. When the patient arrives at the field infirmary, he is laid down, with head low, until he recovers himself. The restoration is left to nature; cold water may be dashed into the face, but all stimulation should be avoided unless the pulse is found to flag, when a little brandy may be cautiously given. The surgeon takes advantage of the insensibility of the patient, shaves the head at the point of injury, and gives the wound a thorough examination. When reaction has taken place, and the patient is restored to consciousness, should the wound have been a simple one of the soft parts, the cold water dressings is all that will be required, and should be applied according to general principles. The thin, wet compress, with oiled or waxed cloth should cover the wound and head for some distance around the injury, and instead of tying these in place by the roll of bandage, the better plan is to adopt the head net of the Prussian medical service. It is a round piece of coarse netting made of cotton yarn: a string ties under the chin to keep the dressing on, and a drawing string, running around the net, like a purse string, attaches it securely to the head around the temples. This is an admirable dressing for all head injuries, which require light, cool, and efficient applications.

Should the soft parts have been much bruised,

the ice bladder will be required to keep down excessive suppuration. To prevent mischief, all injuries of the head demand rest and quiet, avoidance of stimulants, and abstemious diet. By adopting this course in uncomplicated wounds, whether gunshot or sabre, a speedy cure is usually obtained. Effusions of blood under the skin should not be interfered with; incisions are not required. If the effusions are allowed to remain excluded from air, the cold water dressings with arnica will cause their rapid absorption; if the skin is punctured and air admitted, suppuration will surely ensue. Should suppuration occur, as soon as pus can be clearly detected, let it out by a small incision. If this be neglected at the proper time, the pent-up pus will separate the periosteum from the skull, and cause, perhaps, a necrosis of the bones. When suppuration has been well established, an oiled cloth is substituted for water dressings by many surgeons, although the growing disposition is to continue the water dressings until cicatrization is completed.

When the skull has been fractured by a ball, sabre blow, or fragment of shell, the treatment should in no material respect differ from the course pursued in a simple scalp wound. A simple or compound fracture of the skull, uncomplicated with injury to the brain or its meninges, should be managed according to the ordinary principles of surgery, remembering always, however, that the brain is in near proximity, and may have been injured, although no symptoms are present for detecting such a lesion. If the patient is insensible, we adopt the means already recommended for removing shock, viz: place the body in a horizontal posture, and leave the case pretty much to nature—avoiding everything tending to internal stimulation. Whilst insensible, we examine the wound thoroughly, using the finger as a probe; and if any loose speculæ of bone be felt quite free in the wound unconnected with the soft parts, they should be removed. If attached, they must be left to escape spontaneously after suppuration is established.

Gunshot fractures are usually distinctly limited to the portion struck, and seldom ramify as do fractures from diffused blows. It is this concentration of the force within a small compass, and the extended injury to the inner tablet of the skull, which render gunshot injuries of the head so serious. When we are satisfied, from a careful examination of the condition of the bones, that they remain in their normal position without depression, the head is shaved and the wound carefully closed with a strip of adhesive plaster, so as to exclude air. As soon as the patient has revived, the cold water or ice treatment is at once instituted. Should there have been but little shock from the injury, these wet applications should be commenced with on the battle field.

When the patient is put to bed (which should be as soon as possible, for early treatment is all-important), his head and shoulders should be elevated; quiet and absolute rest should be strictly enjoined; the room should be darkened; all stimuli, including light and noise, should be avoided; the bowels should be freely opened by a saline, mercurial, or aloetic cathartic; and for a few days, abstemious diet prescribed. These precautions are necessary to prevent irritation of the brain, with subsequent congestion, inflammation, and effusion. If the patient appears irritable and peevish, without heat of head or fulness of pulse, give opium to quiet him.

The case should be watched with care, and if symptoms of congestion of the brain threaten, with injection of the face, red eyes, hot skin, forcible throbbing of the carotids, increasing headache, with an early tendency to delirium, the patient should be at once bled, the head should be shaved, and an ice bladder be assiduously applied over the entire scalp; the intestines should be freely acted upon for the revulsive effect upon the brain, and for a similar reason, sinapisms should be applied to the legs and thighs. Should relief not be promptly obtained, leeches or cups might be applied to the mastoid processes. Calomel was formerly the universal prescription for threatening cerebral inflammation. Salivation was induced as early as possible, and when the system was brought under its influence, the patient was considered comparatively safe. In modern surgery, calomel has lost its high position, and the dependence upon its salivating powers is annually diminishing. Many still administer it, but not with the confidence of former times.

Should this threatened inflammation not subside under this course of treatment, but after a period of high febrile excitement the delirium becomes merged into stupor, with noisy breathing, dilated pupils, slow, labored pulse, relaxed sphincters and paralysis, the case indicates compression from effusion, within or upon the brain, and chances for life become very doubtful. Perhaps, a thick layer of lymph may have formed upon the cerebral surface, or a quantity of serous fluid collected in the ventricles, or a circumscribed or diffused abscess in or upon the brain. This lymphy effusion sometimes covers the entire surface of one or both hemispheres. The arachnoidal membrane appears to be the one chiefly inflamed. It is thickened, semi opaque, adherent to the brain surface, and reddened in patches. The pia mater and brain substance is highly injected.

If, with the occurrence of these symptoms, the patient be seized with chills, the scalp wound becoming dry, and the tissues puffy, or a collection forms under the periosteum, lifting this membrane from the bones which appear dry and yellow, it would indicate, in many instances, a circumscribed collection of pus within the skull. These symptoms might be, but very rarely are, relieved by the use of the trephine. As a general rule, the operation hastens the fatal catastrophy. Unless an external abscess, with the characteristic puffy scalp, defines the collection of effusions within, the trephine should not be used. It often happens after trephining, that these supposed collections have not been found, and it is only after the operation that the secretion of pus has been established. When air is admitted, suppuration is certain; whilst without the operation the effusions are known, in many instances, to have been absorbed—the patient recovering after remaining insensible, in one case, as long as twenty-one days.

Cole, in his Military Surgery, mentions cases of fracture of the skull from ball, without the skin being torn. Unless the bones are much detached, as they were in one of his cases, the condition can only be suspected. Such injuries must be treated under the antiphlogistic expectant plan. *Await symptoms before active surgical interference is instituted, and we will never regret it.*

There are a series of cases, in which injury to the skull is complicated with internal bleeding. The insensibility which seized the patient at the moment of injury will pass off, and the consciousness will be regained, but only for a time. The patient, after a longer or shorter interval, feels heavy and dull, and indisposed to exertion; finally, a strong disposition to sleep comes over him, which, deepening into coma, ends in all the symptoms of well marked compression. This is an instance in which the surgeons, of twenty years since, would have trephined, as the only chance of saving the patient. Now, we would lay down an equally broad rule, that his only hope of recovery is in avoiding the trephine. Pursue a rigid antiphlogistic course; free venesection, when assisted by ice bladders to the entire scalp, will stop further loss of blood, reduce the action of the heart, and permit the effused blood to clot, so as to close the openings in the torn blood-vessels; then, by free purgation, act upon the bowels, both for a derivative effect, and to promote the absorption of the effusion. If you can stop the further escape of blood, that which has been effused will gradually be removed, and the symptoms of compression will as gradually pass off, after having continued for days, or even weeks. Trephine such a patient, and what certainty have we that we will find the point where hemorrhage has taken place, or that the blood is still fluid, and can be removed—both very improbable results. Blood-vessels may have given way at any other portion of the brain than at the portion corresponding to the point where the skull is injured. The recoil of the contents of the skull may have ruptured vessels diametrically opposite to the injured point. Autopsies not unusually reveal such conditions.

The operation of trephining is always very serious *per se*, and is sufficient of itself to cause cerebral or meningeal inflammation, which will nearly always terminate fatally. The operation is often more serious than the condition for which it is used, and, although the patient might recover from either, he succumbs under the combination. Experience and autopsies have shown us many cases of extensive intra-cranial hemorrhages, which have been unaccompanied by symptoms denoting such an accident; and the traces of such have been found when the patient, recovering from his head injury, had fallen a victim to some totally foreign disease. Had such a condition been suspected, and the surgeon used his instruments, an autopsy at a much earlier day would have revealed the condition.

The third variety of injury of the head, with depression of the skull, belongs to a more serious class of wounds. The complication is detected at once by examining the wound with the finger, when the sinking of the bones is felt, the extent of injury is detected, and the condition of the depressed portion, whether *en masse* or spiculated, determined. The broken fragments, if quite loose, should be removed within the first twenty-four hours, before reaction sets in. When concussion has passed off, and no symptoms exist indicating injurious pressure upon the brain, the case should be treated in every respect as if no depressed fragments existed. Unless we see clearly that the bone is very much spiculated, and that sharp fragments are piercing the meninges, avoid all instrumental interference, even to dilating the wound, for the purpose of facilitating a more accurate diagnosis.

We should never be anxious to see the symptoms of concussion rapidly disappear; let nature abide her time; watch the case and see that the patient suffers no detriment. Examine frequently the pulse, but not the head, and as long as it sustains itself, everything is working to the advantage of the wounded. By rapid reaction torn blood-vessels may not have had time to become plugged up, and internal hemorrhage, which is always serious, might ensue. As soon as the pulse commences to improve, then we commence cold applications, which, if assiduously applied, may prevent the after-venesection. When bloodletting is required, it is preferable to bleed moderately from a large opening, to be repeated, if necessary. The object is to obtain its sedative and revulsive effect, and to despoil to as limited an extent as possible. If from six to ten ounces, from a large opening in the vein, will produce a sensible feeling of faintness, do not draw from sixteen to twenty. This sedative effect might be sustained by leeches or cups to the neck, and by small doses of tart. emetic, veratrum viride, or digitalis—never, however, pushing these remedies to vomiting, which, by tending to congestion of the head, would act injuriously. Revulsives to the intestines, as recommended in the treatment of simple fractures, with ice to the head, are the remedies upon which most reliance is to be placed. Free purgation is not desirable, as the frequent change of position would be injurious to the patient. Should the integuments and pericranium inflame with much swelling, pain and tension, with febrile reaction, incisions, or rather scarifications, may be made to release the pent-up fluids. These, if possible, should be made at a distance from the seat of fracture—the object being to protect the injured bones from atmospheric influences.

Surgeons are now becoming familiar with the fact that considerable depression may exist in the external tablet of the skull without the internal being fractured—the external layer being driven into and condensed within the diploe. Also, that both tablets may be depressed, compressing the brain, without causing harm at any subsequent period. Observation has multiplied these cases to such an extent as to modify the entire treatment of head injuries. Although the cranial cavity is filled with brain, its contents are continually undergoing changes from the excessive vascularity of the brain substance, and, also, from the free communication which exists between the fluid filling the ventricles and the veinous plexus which abound in the brain. By diminishing the blood and water in the brain, accommodation can be made for the depressed bone. As a general rule, in gunshot wounds, with depression of fragments, no remarkable symptoms exhibit themselves, until there is a determination of blood to the head from reaction, from mental or bodily excitement. Rational practice would lead us to combat the tendency to congestion by rest, quiet, cold revulsives and venesection, rather than by the trephine, which experience has shown to be so unprofitable. Opium is now used with much greater freedom in the treatment of injuries of the head than formerly and, when administered with discretion, will, to a certain extent, take the place of trephining. Whenever the patient is restless, sleepless, and irritable with delirium, should the face not be red, nor head hot, it can be used with safety and benefit.

When suppuration is established in the wound, and granulations commence to form, those portions of bone which cannot be saved, will gradually become detached and will escape. A tendency to bleeding in the granulations of the wound is an indication that the fragments of bone have become loose and are ready to be removed. This symptom, which is a valuable one, must be noted.

The fourth variety of injury to the head, where a compound fracture, with depressed fragments, is connected with symptoms of compression, is a very serious accident, and is the only variety of complicated head wound in which surgeons consider instrumental interference called for. Even in this instance, the propriety of trephining is doubted by many of large experience, although no doubt exists that, in some cases, immediate relief has followed the lifting of the depressed bone. It is said, that the successful treatment of such cases will depend more upon the condition of the brain and membranes than merely upon the depression. Should these be lacerated, or in any way injured, inflammation will sooner or later show itself. The operation of trephining, under such circumstances, would increase the local irritation, expose the injured tissues to injurious atmospheric influences, and hasten on a violent and usually fatal inflammation.

If the brain and membranes be not injured,

then it is said that the brain will soon become accustomed to the pressure, and, although insensibility may continue for hours, days, or, as in many instances of ultimate recovery, for weeks, the symptoms of compression will gradually pass off. By not using instruments, the surgeon has the satisfaction of knowing that he has not increased the local trouble by a serious operation. The removal of the symptoms of compression being very gradual, excessive reaction is not likely to follow, and as no air has been admitted to the effusions beneath the skull, the probability of suppuration will be much diminished. When effusions have taken place, the depressed bone acts as a covering, excluding air with its injurious chemical influences. Fluids, uncontaminated by decomposition, can be absorbed. When the skull is opened, and the free admission of air is permitted, suppuration, with, perhaps, pyæmia, is prone to occur.

Stromyer, who is one of the highest authorities on gunshot wounds of the head, and who, as surgeon-in-chief of the Schleswig-Holstein army, had every facility for studying his favorite branch of surgery, gives us as the result of his experience, observation and study, that the trephine can be abandoned in military surgery. In a supplement to his work on Military Surgery, recently published, he states, "*that in military surgery trephining is never needed.*—When the case is so severe as to require the trephine in gunshot wounds, the patient will die in spite of it."—In the last two campaigns, in which he had charge of the army, he has not trephined. Loeffler, a distinguished surgeon in the Prussian service, who has published one of the best books of instruction for military surgeons, after acknowledging Stromyer as the master in all relating to the treatment of gunshot wounds of the head, endorses his views in opposition to trephining.

McLeod gives the following as the Crimean experience:—"As to the use of the trephine—the cases and time for its application—less difference of opinion, I believe, exists among the experienced army surgeons than among civilians; and I think the decided tendency among them is to endorse the modern 'treatment by expectancy,' and to avoid operating except in rare cases. In this, I believe they judge wisely; for when we examine the question carefully, we find that there is not one single indication for having recourse to operations, which cannot, by the adduction of pertinent cases, be shown to be often fallacious." Hewett, in a series of lectures on injuries of the head, published in the Medical Times and Gazette for 1859, which form the most complete treatise extant on the subject, is equally adverse to the trephine. Guthrie, Cole, and Williamson, in their reports, equally confirm the dangers of the trephine, and the great fatality accompanying its use.

The entire records of the science may be searched in vain, to find a duplicate series of successful cases to that reported by Stromyer. Of forty-one cases of fracture, with depression from gunshot wounds, in many of which it was probable that the brain and membranes were injured, only seven died—all the rest recovered. In only *one* case was there any operative interference, *although signs of secondary compression appeared in several.* The antiphlogistic treatment, carefully carried out, was alone adhered to.

No surgeon can doubt that the operation of trephining has cost many a man his life, and although many cases have recovered after the operation, it is a question whether, in the majority of cases, more rapid recovery would not have been obtained without it.

When symptoms of compression ensue in the course of treatment, continue the steady, onward use of antiphlogistic remedies. At this juncture, many surgeons recommend calomel pushed to salivation, which some state to be synonymous with salvation. There is no unanimity, however, on this head; the modern tendency is to treat such cases without the use of mercury.

When balls penetrate or perforate the cranium, the detached piece of bone is driven before the ball into the substance of the brain. The resistance which the ball meets changes its course, and glancing from the depressed fragment, it takes a different direction, burying itself in the brain at some distance from the piece of bone. In by far the majority of cases, death is instantaneous, or soon follows the receipt of injury. There are, nevertheless, a few exceptions to this rule, in which the patient, recovering from the shock and sequelæ, has carried the ball or other missile in his brain for years; and, eventually dying of some disease unconnected with the head, an autopsy reveals the ball embedded in the brain, and surrounded by a mass of lymph. Of ninety-one cases of penetrating and perforating gunshot wounds of the head which were admitted into hospital in the Crimea, all, without exception, proved fatal.

When the openings are examined, it will be found that the hole made in the outer tablet is more or less smooth, whilst the orifice in the inner tablet is much more extensively fractured, and usually much spiculated. This condition of the orifices is owing more to the direction of the blow than from any supposed brittleness in the inner tablet; for, should the ball traverse from within outward, the reversed condition is found. It would be folly to attempt the search after such foreign bodies for the purpose of removing them, as such a piece of meddlesome surgery would ensure a fatal issue, whatever hope of recovery might have been entertained. We have heard of such an instance, where a physician had probed the brain with a silver probe to find a ball, but hope never to see such a piece of barbarous ignorance.

Cole, in his Indian Reports, mentions "that there are many soldiers now doing duty in our ranks, for whom (having been wounded in their heads during the late war) the medical officers had not the smallest hope; and every military surgeon, who has had much practice in the field, has learned not to despair so long as life remains." The thorough probing of such cases, to satisfy the curiosity of a surgeon, would soon have destroyed all hope with the life of the patient.

The general treatment of such cases should, in no wise, differ from that laid down for the treatment of head injuries in general. The concussion and compression, which are well marked and always present, must be met with all the precautions already pointed out.

We might now sum up, in a few words, the rational and successful treatment of gunshot wounds of the head. In concussion, unless there is evident sinking, leave the case to nature, and avoid, studiously, both stimulation and venesection. When the patient is restored to consciousness, should inflammation of the brain threaten, if there be no congestion of the face, give opium to allay irritation. Should congestion be evident, use the antiphlogistic treatment locally and generally, commencing with venesection, and with ice applications to the head. In every case, absolute quiet and rest are essential. For the want of a proper sentinel at the door of the ward in which head injuries are being treated, many cases have been lost. All gunshot injuries of the head are serious, however trivial they may appear, inasmuch as violent inflammation often follows slight wounds; all, therefore, should be carefully watched.

Chronic ostitis or periostitis, resulting from gunshot wounds, possesses no peculiarity, and should be combated by iodide of potassium.

CHAPTER VIII.

Wounds of the Face—Fractures of the upper and lower jaw—Wounds of the neck—Large vessels avoid the perforating ball—When large arteries in the neck are divided, the necessity of ligating the bleeding mouths.

Wounds of the Face, when they do not implicate the brain, are not usually of a serious character. The severe cuts about the face, made by the sabre or by pieces of shell, should be treated for adhesion by the first intention. The lips should be brought together by sutures, and cold water dressings will complete the cure. The excessive swelling, which accompanies many injuries of the face, especially gunshot wounds and burns from explosion of powder, is rarely controlled by cold water dressings. It runs its harmlesss course, moderated by the cold applications, and subsides at the end of a few days. In the Itálian campaign, I saw cases in which Minnié balls had traversed the breadth of the face, passing through each molar bone, without leaving any injurious sequelæ. The rapidity with which all wounds of the face heal has often been remarked.

The most common injuries to the face from gunshot wounds are fractures of the upper and lower jaws. Balls often become embedded in the soft, spongy bones of the face, and, if not discovered in time, are discharged spontaneously. When the bones of the face are struck by a grape-shot, or a flattened conical ball, there may be great destruction of the features, followed by shocking deformity.

The senses are not unfrequently destroyed—sight or smell being often impaired, if not completely lost after gunshot injuries. Where the wound has been received in the orbit, the loss of vision is not only very probable, but there is great fear that the cause producing the injury, whether it be a ball, bayonet, or a sword point, may have perforated the thin plate of the skull, entered the brain and may induce cerebral inflammation. Many cases of apparently trivial wounds of the eyelids have terminated fatally, and an autopsy revealed serious injury to the anterior lobes of the brain and its enveloping membranes. Such cases should be carefully watched, and any cerebral symptoms, which may arise, should be actively met by the antiphlogistic treatment, headed by venesection.

From the great vascularity of all the structures composing the face, we would expect to have serious hemorrhage accompanying all injuries—for controlling which, the astringents of iron will be frequently required. The vessels are so numerous that the direct application of ligatures cannot be made. In fractures of the upper jaw, the bones are always more or less spiculated, with one or more teeth loosened or completely detached. As all portions are freely supplied with blood-vessels, union will take place among the fragments, even after considerable shattering of the bones. Unless the fragments are either completely detached or but slightly adherent, they should not be taken away, but should be replaced with care, as, in time, consolidation may take place and very little permanent deformity will be left. Should some of these fragments die, they will be found loose, often as early as the sixth or eighth day, and should be removed. The cold water dressings, to relieve the excessive swelling, with an occasional dose of salts, is the only medication required. The wound in the face should be closed with adhesive plaster, and, after careful adjustment of the movable fragments, and the use of cold water dressings for a few days, the case is left pretty much to nature.

When the soft parts, as well as the bones, are crushed, secondary hemorrhage frequently recurs, as the sloughing tissues come away. Formerly, the difficulty of restraining this loss of blood was so great as to require, in many cases, the ligation of the main vessels in the neck. We now find the thorough application of the per-chloride or per-sulphate of iron an efficient remedy. Should necrosis follow injuries to the bones of the face, the dead pieces of bone should be removed as they become loosened, or a special operation may be undertaken for ridding the face of the local cause of trouble.

Fractures of the lower jaw are not a rare accident on the battle field, whether from shot wounds or other accidents. At times, the entire jaw may be swept off by a round shot, leaving the mouth and throat exposed. One of the most fearful cases on record is one in which the entire face was carried away by a cannon ball, leaving nothing but the skull proper, appended to the vertebral column. The opened gullet marked the former site of the features. The patient lived ten hours, and from the frequent change of position, and the squeezing of the hand when his was taken, it was thought that consciousness remained up to the time of death.

The surgeon accompanying the transport usually sends injuries of the face to the field infirmary untouched, or, should the lower jaw be broken, applies a folded handkerchief or band under it to support it. It is permanently put up in a paste-board splint, well padded with carded cotton, and secured by a folded cloth or double-tailed bandage. One band passes over the vertex, supporting the jaws, whilst the other passes from the front of the chin behind the head, and then around the forehead, where it is secured by pins. Before the dressings are applied, the wounds should have been examined carefully with the finger, and all perfectly-detached spiculæ of bone should have been removed. The surgeon must be prepared to meet much swelling and profuse salivation. All wounds of the bones of the face being compound, suppuration is soon established, and the secretion of pus is copious. It will add much to the comfort of the patient if his mouth be swabbed out daily with a piece of soft rag or sponge attached to a thin piece of wood. From the difficulty in swallowing, fluid nourishment must be prescribed. The constant thirst of those wounded will be relieved by small doses of morphine, or by acidulated drinks, made either with diluted nitric acid or vinegar. Injuries about the face are very liable to erysipelatous attacks. The treatment by the tincture of the muriate of iron, locally and generally, will stop its progress.

Wounds of the neck, with injury to the numerous large vessels which course through this constricted region, are among the serious accidents in battle. From the anatomy of this region, we would suppose that a missile could not traverse the neck in any direction without destroying some important part, nerve or artery. We find, after every great battle, perforations by balls in every direction, accompanied by violent hemorrhages; yet, with the first fainting brought on from shock and loss of blood, we find a spontaneous cessation of the bleeding, and the onward progress of the case becomes one of continued convalescence, to perfect cicatrization. I have seen conical balls perforate the neck antero-posteriorly, entering just above the sterno-clavicular junction, and passing in the midst, if not through, the largest vessels of the body, without producing a fatal hemorrhage. I have also seen them perforate the throat laterally, on a level with and just behind the angle of the lower jaw, and a cure equally follow. It is wonderful how the great vessels escape, or the rapidity with which clots form and the wounds of such vessels close. McLeod reports one hundred and twenty-eight cases, more or less severely injured in the neck, with but four deaths. Many, to be sure, die on the battle field in a few moments after receiving a serious injury to the large arteries; but, undoubtedly, many also recover.

The powerful iron styptics are the only local remedies applicable on the battle field, as the patient could not otherwise bear the transportation; and the assistant surgeon, following the troops, has neither the time nor conveniences for ligating the bleeding mouths of the divided vessel, however urgently it may be called for, to save life. The precautions which were urged in discussing the means of arrest of hemorrhage in wounds generally must here be carefully applied; and should secondary hemorrhage occur, and be renewed, notwithstanding the careful application of the iron styptic, the safety of the patient will then lie only in the ligation of both bleeding orifices. The anastomosis is so free in the neck, that all other operations will be futile, and the patient will perish. A ligature upon the carotid artery, both above and below the wound, has been reported a failure in controlling a hemorrhage, which was only checked by dilating the wound and ligating the artery at the point injured. In enlarging the wound, the incision will always be made parallel with the axis of the neck, so as to avoid injuring important nerves or blood-vessels.

CHAPTER IX.

Wounds of the Chest—Flesh wounds—Effusions within the cavity when the pleura is injured—Wounds of the heart or lung — A transfixed chest does not necessarily imply a perforated lung — Diagnostic value of the various symptoms—Hæmoptysis, Dyspnœa, Collapse, Emphysema — Treatment of chest wounds—How inflammatory complications are to be combated—The treatment of a fractured rib.

Wounds of the Chest, when taken as a class, are perhaps the most fatal of gunshot wounds. Many are shot down, and die more or less rapidly on the battle field from internal hemorrhage, with its accompanying suffocation, and are returned among the killed. Fraser, in an excellent treatise on chest wounds, based upon data obtained in the Crimea, states the mortality to have been twenty-eight per cent. of all chest wounds, and seventy-nine per cent. of those in which the lung had been injured. The Russian report gives as their mortality in chest wounds ninety-eight per cent., which is sufficient proof of their serious character. The danger in wounds of the thorax is from visceral complications. Should the lung be severely injured, the case usually terminates fatally.

From the peculiar formation of the thoracic box and the curve of the ribs, balls, in striking, are often deflected from the straight line, and, after a longer or shorter course, escape without having penetrated the chest. Often, the two openings correspond so accurately in direction, as to establish a strong conviction of a direct passage through or across the thorax, when the wound has been but a subcutaneous one throughout. I have seen an instance in which a ball, which had entered the chest just below the left armpit, was removed from a similar position in the right side, and, although it had apparently traversed the thorax, no inconvenience was experienced; its entire course had been subcutanoeus. This tortuous track can only be made by a ball striking at a considerable obliquity. Its direction is generally indicated by a reddish or purplish line under the skin, which, when followed by the finger pressed on the surface, imparts a crackling sensation, caused by air in the cellular tissue. Such injuries are usually simple, and require but little treatment. The cold water dressing fills every indication, and its application for a few days usually effects a cure.

A great amount of nervous shock often accompanies very trivial injuries of the chest. Many instances are mentioned by military surgeons in which balls had struck articles about the person of the soldier — the breast-plate of a cuirassier, or, perhaps, a book in the breast-pocket of a soldier's coat—and had fallen to the ground without even touching the skin, yet the soldier had been knocked down breathless, and, in some cases, did not recover completely from the shock for days.

When the ball has penetrated the chest, it may course for some distance between the ribs and the pleura, when it may either escape from the cavity, and be found under the skin, or remain capped by the pleura. Such cases may give no trouble, or pleuritis may ensue, which the rational signs, with discultation, will detect, and an antiphlogistic course, accompanied with the free use of opium, will readily subdue. Opium, when used in large doses, frequently repeated, possesses other virtues than merely allaying pain and quieting nervous symptoms. It combats, directly, inflammation, and, by the great control which it exercises over the brain and circulation, becomes one of the most, if not the most valuable remedy of the materia medica in the treatment of the serious sequelæ of wounds. When given in combination with nitrate or carb. of soda, its nauseating effects are counteracted.

The evil which the surgeon fears from perforating wounds, followed by inflammation, is that a serous, or sero-purulent effusion may rapidly accumulate in the thoracic cavity, and destroy the patient. So rapidly is this fluid formed, in many cases, that the chest has been known to fill in twenty-four or forty-eight hours, the fluid compressing and condensing the lung against the vertebral column. In expanding the chest, it will be found that as soon as a thin layer of fluid is effused into the cavity, separating the lung from the thoracic wall, the respiratory murmur becomes very feeble, and will altogether disappear when the cavity is filled. At the same time respiration becomes much embarrassed with marked dyspnœa. Percussing the side, will now give a dull, heavy sound, instead of the ordinary clear, sonorous one of health; and the position of the patient, unless the cavity is filled with fluid, must vary the sound by the gravitation of the serous collection. The lung is condensed and flattened against the vertebral column, and is temporarily impervious to air: under a long continuance of the pressure, it will become permanently consolidated. The increase in the circumference of the chest, and the fulness of the intercostal spaces, and the absence to a great extent of respiratory movements upon the affected side, are conspicuous symptoms of a distended cavity.

The quantity of fluid thrown out varies from a few ounces to several pints. When the natural dimensions of the cavity are not sufficiently extensive to accommodate it, it forces the mediastinum over to the sound side, interfering with the action of the healthy lung, whilst an encroachment may be equally made upon the abdomen.

When the surgeon has recognized such collections as rapidly forming in the chest after gunshot wounds, accompanied by distressing symptoms of dyspnœa, an early evacuation will be required. Should the collection be purulent, and show a disposition to point, an opening for the escape of the fluid should be made at the point which nature indicates, but, in cases of excessive effusion, any broad intercostal space, between the sixth and eighth ribs on the right, or between the seventh and ninth on the left, might be the point selected. The instrument, usually a trocar and canula, should be introduced at right angles to the chest and near the upper edge of the rib, toward its angle, in a line continuous with the posterior border of the arm-pit. As this puncture corresponds with the lowest portion of the cavity, the chest can be perfectly drained through it.

In all gunshot injuries of the chest, the serious complication is injury to the lungs or heart, and it is often difficult to detect at first such lesions. Notwithstanding the many infallible signs laid down by authors, military surgeons of experience inform us that no one symptom is sufficient for making a diagnosis. When the heart is injured, although instantaneous death does not takes place as a general rule, the wounded man lives but a short period. The pericardium soon becomes filled with blood; the action of the heart is mechanically impeded, and, sooner or later, depending upon the size of the wound and the facility for letting out blood, it ceases its pulsation. Reports of cases are not very rare in which small, oblique incised wounds of the heart have been recovered from; and even gunshot wounds of this organ, perforating its cavities, have escaped with life. When the pericardium is perforated, and the heart not injured, a successful result might be obtained by a judicious course of antiphlogistic treatment, which will keep down inflammation, with its effusions of lymph and serum.

The lung often escapes injury when, from the position of the wounds of entrance and of exit, with the certainty of the cavity being transfixed, the natural belief would lead to a perforation of the lung. A straight line between the wounds passes apparently through the substance of the lung, but the ball in perforating the rib had been deflected from its straight course, had followed, perhaps, the inner curve of the chest, and, meeting with some resistance, had forced its way through the chest, either appearing under the tough, elastic skin, or escaping without touching the contained organs.

The lung may, on the other hand, be severely injured when no perforating wound exists. A blow by a spent ball, or a fragment of shell, may make a very superficial wound or bruise in the skin, and yet may shatter one or more ribs, driving the spiculæ into the lung, lacerating to a greater or less extent its substance. Even without fracture of the ribs, the concussion or blow may have been sufficiently great to have caused irreparable injury to the lung. The severity of the symptoms will depend upon the depth of the injury in the lung. The deeper the lung is perforated, the larger are the blood-vessels implicated and the more excessive and rapid the hemorrhage. It is on account of this loss that the most conspicuous symptoms arise, viz: hemorrhage, collapse and suffocation.

The patient may be at once suffocated by a large quantity of blood filling up the thorax, and preventing the ingress of air into the lungs. Usually blood passes from both mouth and wound; that from the mouth is frothy and florid, and is brought up by a short, tickling, harassing cough. The size of the dark-colored stream, pouring from the wound, depends upon the position of the orifice. Where the orifice is situated low upon the chest, and is large and direct, the effusion into the cavity escapes freely—the symptoms of collapse may soon appear, but suffocation is prevented; whilst from an injury in the upper portion of the chest, particularly if small and oblique, the thorax may fill with blood, and suffocation becomes imminent, without much external loss. The danger from hemorrhage is greatest during the first twelve hours, and is pretty well over by the second day. It may, however, continue for eight or ten days, gradually diminishing in quantity. With the flow of blood from the wound, air often escapes, and the two symptoms are considered unequivocal proof that the lungs have been injured, although their absence do not prove the contrary.

The mere loss of blood from the lung is no certain indication that the organ has been injured, as bloody expectoration is a common symptom of blows upon the chest, and may accompany the most trivial injury. Fraser, in his recent work on gunshot wounds of the chest, places a less value on hæmoptysis than do other military surgeons. Guthrie considers it a proof of lung wound, so does Baudens, McLeod, Stromyer, Ballingall and others. Fraser's experience in the Crimea, gives, in nine fatal cases in which the lungs were wounded, but one instance of hæmoptysis, and, in seven fatal cases in which the lungs were not injured, two had a spitting of blood. In twelve cases of recovery, three had hæmoptysis. He, therefore, infers that spitting of blood is a very deceptive diagnostic sign of lung wound. When it is rapidly brought up by mouthfuls it becomes an important symptom.

The discharge from the wound is sometimes occasioned by injury to the intercostal vessel, but this is so rarely the case that McLeod states that he neither saw nor heard of an instance during the Crimean war.

The most distressing symptom is dyspnœa, which may appear soon after the injury has been received, or, perhaps, not until some days have intervened; in certain cases of undoubted lung injury it may not have been present at any time. This symptom is sometimes very intense, from moral or other causes, when the lung is not wounded, and it may be but slightly marked, or even altogether absent, when the lung is seriously implicated. This difficulty in breathing depends in some instances upon the direct pressure and condensation of the lung by air or by fluids. When the chest has been opened by a ball, the lung does not collapse as is generally supposed, but, if the opening is sufficiently large, can be seen moving to and fro against the thoracic walls simultaneously with respiration; and, as a proof of the continued action of the lung, and its inflation with air, it is sometimes found protruding from the orifice, forming a hernia of the organ. Even when the lung has been completely perforated, it does not necessarily collapse, but as blood escapes into the pleural cavity, the lung may be driven back and condensed against the vertebral column, with the accompanying symptoms of dyspnœa. From injury to the lung and continued escape of air into the pleural sac, we sometimes find similar difficulties in respiration induced.

Emphysema is a symptom of injury to the lung upon which much importance has been placed. It can occur under any circumstance by which air is admitted into the pleural cavity, where, being compressed by the action of the lung and walls of the chest, it is forced out through the wound; but if a ready exit is not offered for its escape, or should any obstacle exist in the form, size, or direction of the wound, it is forced into the cellular tissue. Owing to the free communication in the interstices of areolar tissues, it diffuses itself widely and rapidly. Should a perforated wound from ball or other weapon allow air to enter the pleural cavity, whether the lung be injured or not, emphysema might appear. It is not so common after gunshot wounds, as a free exit is offered to the contents of the cavity. It is a much more common accompaniment of oblique punctured wounds by sword point or bayonet, and also in cases of fractured ribs, when sharp spiculæ of bone have abraided the surface of the lung and allowed air to escape from the air tubes into the cavity: as it is found either with or without lung injury, it cannot be of much value in diagnosis. The injured lung, in gunshot wounds, does not often permit air to escape for any length of time from its wounded surface, as an immediate extravasation of blood into the bruised tissue closes up the air tubes and shuts off communication with the cavity.

Another symptom of great value is *collapse*, depending upon loss of blood. It is well known that all the blood of the body must continually pass through the lungs, and should the vessels composing the parenchyma of this organ be extensively opened, the loss in even a short period must be excessive. It is not surprising, therefore, that the patient should soon become cold, pale, and faint—with feeble, small and irregular pulse, and with rapid tendency to syncope. This is nature's effort to check further loss; and although sometimes successful, often gives but temporary security. The surgeon tries to induce this condition for a similar purpose.

From consideration of the above symptoms we are induced to believe that no one symptom is pathognomonic of injury to the lung, but it is rather from a combination of phenomena that any certainty in diagnosis is attained. The immediate danger and intensity of the symptoms will depend upon the depth of penetration. Where the chest is only superficially wounded, although the force of the blow may be sufficient to produce an amount of shock of shorter or longer duration, and blood may be expectorated from the concussion of the lungs, the symptoms will be trivial. The pain of the bruised tissues will pass off in a few days, and with it all the accompanying symptoms. When the chest has been opened without injury to the lung, heart, or intercostal vessels, the symptoms are also trivial, and unless inflammation of the pleura and subsequent effusions of serum or pus should ensue, the case will equally require but little treatment. When the lung is implicated, and especially when severely wounded, other symptoms are more or less conspicuously present. Soon after the reception of a severe wound, blood pours from the injured vessels and escapes both into the air tubes and into the pleural cavity.

From the air vessels it is brought up and expectorated, in greater or less quantity as hæmoptysis, whilst it flows from the external wound in the side. If both openings in lung and chest be free, the blood escaping is mingled with air when the patient coughs. With the loss of blood, the surface becomes cold and bedewed with a cold perspiration; the pulse is weak and tremulous, becoming more and more enfeebled until syncope comes on, which temporarily checks the excessive bleeding. Should the orifice in the side offer an imperfect escape to the blood, it collects in the pleural cavity, rapidly encroaches upon the lung, which is forced back against the spinal column, and by compressing the opposite side of the chest through the mediastinum, threatens suffocation. The eyes protrude, nostrils expand to their utmost, the arms are thrown about in every direction, and frightful struggles for breath appear in every feature; these are the cases which, if not immediately relieved, will in a few moments terminate fatally by suffocation.

The field surgeon, in transporting those wounded in the chest, will give the most careful attention to the severely wounded. The simple cases, requiring no immediate attendance, will be sent on to the field infirmary. Although the wound has evidently transfixed the chest, if no urgent symptoms exist, the case is also carefully conveyed to the infirmary, or even directly on to the general hospital; but should the distressing symptoms above mentioned follow soon after the injury has been received, then the life of the patient is in the hands of the ambulance surgeon, and should he ignore or neglect the case, the soldier may not reach the infirmary alive. Notwithstanding the hemorrhage, open a large vein and draw away blood, if possible, to syncope. The safety of the patient depends upon this being obtained; as in the interval, when the heart's action is at its minimum, but little blood will be driven to the lungs, and a disposition to the formation of a clot may plug up the bleeding vessels. The dyspnœa, and not the pulse, will be the indication for bleeding in lung wounds. The patient is not detained on the field to see the effects of the venesection, but, with his vein open, is sent on to the field infirmary, accompanied by the surgeon himself, or by an intelligent assistant. As soon as he faints, the surgeon at the field infirmary removes the rough field dressing, examines the wound with the finger, and, if not sufficiently large to permit a thorough search for foreign bodies, where such are suspected, he dilates it with a probe-pointed bistoury.

In perforating chest wounds, unless urgent symptoms of dyspnœa are present, the general treatment is the expectant plan. The wound having been carefully closed with diachylon, the patient lies on the wounded side, so as to throw the lung against the orifice, hoping that it may adhere to the chest at that point, and so close the cavity; he also finds this the most comfortable position. He is kept quiet, in a dark room; all excitants are avoided, rigid diet is instituted; veratrum viride, or digitalis, is given to control the action of the heart; opium is freely administered to quiet the constant hacking, trickling cough, and iced cloths or bladders are applied to the chest. With such treatment and careful watching, seeing the patient, if possible, every hour, we await the development of symptoms. The accurate closure of the wound excludes the admission of air, and, to a certain extent, prevents emphysema, and also the rapid decomposition of the escaped fluids in the cavity.

If it be a shot wound, with a single orifice, and the clothing be found perforated, the wound should be examined for foreign bodies. If found, extract them; if not detected, then close the wound carefully with a strip of diachylon, and apply the water or ice dressing. The search for foreign bodies must always be made with the finger, and should never be protracted. Should nothing be found after a moderate, intelligent search, close the wound, and await developments. This examination should be made before reaction comes on. Should we not see the patient until he is feverish, all examinations must be absolutely forbidden for at least eight days, until the reaction has subsided and suppuration well established. It is well known that balls, etc., even pieces of clothing, have been found encysted in the lungs years after they had been deposited; and, in some instances, these articles have been expectorated during a severe spell of coughing, after long intervals. Although always desirable that these be removed, a prolonged search may entail such an amount of injury as to destroy all hope of saving the patient, when the presence of the foreign body would not have been necessarily incompatible with life or even health. Besides, when suppuration is well established, we have a second and much better opportunity for a careful examination, without much fear of doing injury.

Should the gradual accumulation of blood in the cavity of the chest cause dyspnœa, the orifice may require opening, to allow the fluid to escape and relieve the pressure upon the lung. In drawing off the contents of the chest, if syncope threatens, we close the opening, and await another opportunity. The collection is retained in certain cases, when no dyspnœa exists, for the purpose of retarding, and finally controlling the bleeding, by pressure upon the lung and its injured blood-vessels. After the third or fourth day, the tendency to hemorrhage having ceased, and the wound having already commenced to suppurate, the adhesive plaster is removed, and the effusion is allowed to escape. If air has been admitted into the cavity, the exuded blood has decomposed and, mingled with serum and pus, makes a copious and very offensive discharge for the first few days. Gradually the escaping fluid loses its dark color and offensive smell, and assumes the appearance of healthy pus. Formerly much care was taken to favor the flow of fluids from the chest, and dilatation of the wound was the recognized rule; now, the opposite treatment is the one urged to exclude air, and if possible, retard decomposition, as this deterioration of the effused fluids is more injurious to the system than the advantages obtained by their ready escape. From this time onward, simple water dressing will be the only local treatment required for the wound. If the orifice from a punctured wound has healed, with escaped blood remaining within the chest, the collection, if small, should be ignored, as it will gradually be absorbed; but if the extravasation be extensive, particularly if air had previously entered the cavity, it must be withdrawn through a puncture made at the most dependant portion of the chest. This operation, unless called for by urgent or distressing symptoms, should never be hastily performed, but should, on the contrary, be delayed as long as possible.

During the treatment of perforating wounds of the chest, dyspnœa, whenever urgent, should always be removed by the lancet, the venesection to be repeated as frequently as called for by threatened suffocation, unless this symptom be clearly traced to pent-up fluid, when opening the wound or enlarging it, to permit a ready escape, will remove the oppression of breathing. Prompt and repeated venesection will also be required to control hemorrhage, which is a common cause of death in such injuries, and will alone diminish the number of victims of chest wounds. In collapse, we have already recognized a valued aid for checking hemorrhage, and its remediable advantages should be appreciated. As a symptom, it must be carefully watched, and should it threaten to stop the action of the heart, external stimulation must be freely used, but the internal stimuli must be administered only in small quantity and with great caution. When the immediate dangers have passed, the next in order is inflammation of the lung and pleura. Neither of these conditions differ in any very material respect from the idiopathic varieties of the disease. The traumatic pneumonia is sometimes circumscribed to narrow limits, and its cause may, to a certain extent, modify the general symptoms. As the cause of pleuritis is a direct injury to the membrane, and, in the majority of instances, as air has been admitted within the cavity, the effusions which accompany the inflammation soon become purulent, and in time false membranes of considerable thickness line the inner surface of the ribs. The treatment for either pneumonia or pleurisy, when occurring from a gunshot wound, does not differ from the treatment of the disease from any other cause. McLeod's experience is in favor of early, active, and repeated bleedings, with cool drink and abstemious diet, recognizing, at the same time, however, that many excellent recoveries have been made without recourse to the lancet. Guthrie uses the lancet, which he designates the first and most essential remedy, and which he says should be resorted to in every case. The venesection, which he repeats whenever the inflammatory symptoms show an increase, is vigorously followed by large doses of tartar emetic in pneumonia, and calomel in pleurisy, the object being to affect the gums as soon as possible. This is the treatment of the old school, which recent experience does not uphold. Guthrie states "that in the Crimea bloodletting had not been so favorably viewed, nor found so serviceable, nor so necessary." Fraser, from Crimean experience, states that in the prevention and reduction of inflammatory action in perforating wounds of the chest, venesection is not demanded. It should only be used when the pulse is full, strong, and labored—a condition not often met with. When the heart and pulse are both weak, a common condition after severe wounds, the abstraction of blood will occasion a complete prostration of strength, and may be fatal.

There is no reason for changing the plan of treatment, already discussed in detail, for combating inflammation following gunshot wounds, and which is equally applicable to chest wounds. Even when the lung is inflamed we would prefer the mild, expectant and antiphlogistic treatment to the spoliative. Absolute rest, cooling beverages, moderate nourishment, avoiding over-stimulation, with small doses of tart. emetic, veratrum or digitalis, with the liberal use of opium, and attention to the intestinal secretions, will be required in all cases, and in many will compose the entire treatment.

A certain degree of pleuritis is expected and desired in penetrating lung wounds, to establish adhesions between the injured lung and thoracic wall, which will at once isolate the injured portion and prevent inflammatory sequelæ. As gunshot wounds do not close rapidly but usually suppurate, permitting the free access of air within the thorax, the suppuration will be profuse and long-continued. We must remember this in the treatment, and not use depressing agents. When the pleuritis is excessive and general, both false membranes and the rapid accumulation of fluid are to be anticipated. If the external wound is still open, the position of the body, which is very important, will allow the ready escape of the effusion, which is, at first, serous, but soon becomes purulent. Position and constitutional support will form the basis of treatment. If the pus could have a constant outlet for escape, and accumulation within the cavity could be prevented, the false membranes would tie the lung to the thoracic wall at a much earlier period, and, by obliterating the pleural cavity, prevent further discharge. Should the wound be in the upper portion of the chest, it would hasten the cure to establish a counter-opening from the most dependant portion of the cavity, from which the drain would never be interrupted.

The chapter on the treatment of suppurating wounds lays down general laws for counteracting the injurious influences of long-continued suppuration. Penetrating wounds of the thorax occasionally remain fistulous for an almost indefinite period, which is caused by a failure of general adhesion between the costal and pulmonary pleuræ. A kind of pouch is found, lined by a false membrane, from which a purulent lymph is continually secreted. After empyema, the chest contracts, the walls sink in, the diaphragm rises high on the affected side, the spine becomes contorted, air enters indifferently into the lung, little or no respiratory movements are seen in the chest, and a portion of the respiratory apparatus is rendered useless to the economy. Usually, the long train of symptoms terminate fatally in phthisis. Very few cases of injury to the lung, from gunshot wounds, are ever restored to health.

In cases of fractured ribs, from gunshot injuries, the bone is usually spiculated, and some of the fragments may accompany the ball in its onward course. Upon examination with the finger—executed with great caution from the fear of pushing the fragments into the chest and converting a simple wound into a perforating wound, always a serious accident—these irregular fragments, if detected, should be removed, and, if necessary, the outer wound should be enlarged to facilitate this important step. The danger is not so much from the breaking of the bone, but from the displaced, sharp fragments, which may seriously injure the pleuræ and lung. When removed, and the sharp edges of the rib, which turn in toward the cavity, are excised, the wound should be closed with a wide, adhesive strap, and cold water dressings applied. If no symptoms indicate injury to the lung, a broad band may surround the chest, to control the thoracic movements and allay the pain; but, should any oppression in the breathing show itself, the bandage cannot be applied, as it will increase the suffocative feelings. Where the spiculæ are not displaced, a broad adhesive strap is the only local apparatus required. Necrosis of the rib very commonly follows a gunshot fracture, and may require a subsequent resection for its removal.

When an intercostal artery is divided, the bleeding point will be discovered by drawing out the lips of the wound with a tenaculum, when the vessel should be secured. All military surgeons agree that this operation is more frequently spoken of than performed. Many of extensive experience have never seen a case.

When foreign bodies, as balls, pieces of bone, cloth, wadding, etc., are driven into the pleural cavity they produce fatal results, by inflammation and exhausting discharges, unless removed. A loose ball can be sometimes felt by the patient, and its movements often detected by the stethescope. Through an opening, made at the most dependant portion of the chest, the foreign body can be removed successfully.

CHAPTER X.

Wounds of abdomen—Flesh wounds—Never probe perforating wounds of the abdomen, and, especially, never attempt to search for foreign bodies which have passed beyond the abdominal walls—Sew up intestinal wounds—Dilate wound in abdomen when necessary to relieve strangulation and facilitate reduction—Where the larger viscera are injured, recovery is rare—Avoid using purgatives when the intestine is wounded—Peritonitis a common cause of mortality—Where the intestine is much crushed, leave it out of the wound, or excise the crushed portion and close the intestinal wound by sutures—In wounds of the bladder, continued use of catheter essential.

Sir Charles Bell has remarked that, although *abdominal wounds* bore a fair relative proportion to other wounds, immediately after a battle, a few days sufficed to remove them—so that, by the end of the first week, there was scarcely one to be seen. As a rule, all who have received wounds of the large abdominal viscera die—the exception, of restoration to health, being rarely met with. Like wounds of the chest, where the abdominal walls are not perforated, but the entire track of the ball lies in the thickness of the muscles, the wound is simply a flesh wound and should be treated accordingly. The track of the ball is not always in a straight course, as the muscles, or their tendinous portions, when in action, offer sufficient resistance to turn the ball. The fascia transversalis is said to show a similar resistance to oblique shot.

A perforating wound of the abdomen is equally dangerous as those of the chest, from the fear of peritonitis, which is apt to supervene. If the perforation be made by a sword or bayonet, or if there be any prospect of healing by the first intention, the wound should be accurately closed by adhesive straps or by sutures. In sewing up an abdominal wound, many recommend that the needle should not pass deeper than the superficial cellular tissue, giving as a reason that when the muscles are included in the sutures, they sometimes draw themselves out of the noose by their contraction, whilst, if the peritoneum be also included, peritonitis is much more likely to occur. Although this may hold good for the peritoneum, I can see no reason why attempts should not be made to cause union in the muscles, and, therefore, avoiding the peritoneum, I would include all the tissues, even to the transversalis fascia, in the suture. When this is done, the cicatrix will be firmer, and there will be less probability of secondary hernia—a very common accident after injury to the abdominal walls.

In probing abdominal wounds, the only object to be sought by the examination is whether the wound has perforated or not. From the direction of the track this can nearly always be determined. As in any other gunshot wound, the use of the silver probe is very dangerous, as it may convert a simple into a perforating wound; whilst with the finger, or a gum bougie, the course of the wound, should it be a flesh wound, can be traced, and also the existence of foreign bodies detected. Should we find that the opening transfixes the abdominal wall, our examination should go no further—it is a dangerous amusement to satisfy curiosity at the expense of such irreparable mischief as may destroy the life of the patient.

If the wound be a large one, as when made by a sabre-bayonet, fragment of shell, or Minnié ball, a portion of the abdominal contents may protrude from the wound. When the ambulance surgeon finds such a case on the field, his first duty will be to examine the protrusion. If it be a portion of small intestine and be not injured, he cleanses it of dirt and all other extraneous substances, by pouring water upon it, and carefully returning it within the abdomen, closes the wound by sutures, if it be an incised wound; or a broad strip of diachylon plaster, if a gunshot wound. He then administers a dose of morphine, and sees that the wounded man is properly transported to the field infirmary. To facilitate the return of the protrusion, whether it be intestinal or omental, the patient is placed upon his back with the thighs drawn up, and the abdominal muscles relaxed, when the ambulance surgeon makes steady pressure upon the protrusion in the direction of the wound. The bowel must be handled very carefully—no force should be used, or so much injury might be inflicted as to cause the rupture, sloughing or inflammation of the protruding organ. The better plan would be to encircle the protrusion by the fingers clustered together as a funnel or cone, which will diminish the bulk at the opening in the abdomen, and facilitate its return. If it be found that the mass is so constricted by the small size of the orifice, that the return within the abdominal cavity is impossible without inflicting injury upon the bowel, the intestine should be drawn to one side, and, using great caution, the wound should be enlarged upward for a quarter or half an inch. As the constriction is rarely in the peritoneal wound but usually in the muscles and fascia, the incision, if possible, should not include the peritoneum. Cutting upon a grooved director, or using a probe-pointed bistoury, will diminish the dangers of wounding important parts within whilst enlarging the wound. The return of the bowel should always be effected by the ambulance surgeon before the case is transported to the field infirmary, inasmuch as the crowding of the wounded at the infirmary may be such that several hours might elapse between the receipt of injury and the hospital examination—quite long enough to cause strangulation of the intestine, and either necessitate inflammation or mortification of the protrusion, usually a fatal complication in abdominal wounds. The early return of the protruding intestine makes the case one for simple and successful treatment. Be satisfied that the intestine has been returned within the abdominal cavity, and not forced under the sheaths of the abdominal muscles, where it would strangulate and rapidly destroy life.

Should the case not be seen until several hours had elapsed, the intestine should be equally returned whether it be congested or inflamed; but when gangrenous, which is recognized by its greenish ash color, loss of polish, its flaccid condition, with already a disposition to separation in its various coats, it should remain without the wound, and be laid open so as to allow its fecal contents to be evacuated. Adhesions rapidly form, uniting the protruded intestine to the peritoneum at the inner orifice of the wound. This shuts off all connection with the peritoneal cavity, and prevents extravasation of fecal matter within it. If the bowel be returned in a mortified condition, the contents of the bowel would be discharged into the peritoneal cavity, and fatal peritonitis would be excited.

Should the intestine be injured, it is left in situ, covered with a wet or oiled cloth, until the wounded soldier reaches the field infirmary, when it is closed with one, two, or more points of interrupted suture, according to the size of the opening—a stitch being placed for every one-sixth of an inch of intestinal wound. The ends of the suture are cut off close to the knot, and the whole is returned into the abdomen with care. A fine cambric needle will be the best instrument for sewing up intestinal wounds, as the small puncture and fine thread produce scarcely any irritation. In passing the sutures, do not include the lining mucus membrane in the noose, for if this be allowed to pout between the lips of the intestinal wound it might interfere with rapid healing; the serous or peritoneal layers should be brought in contact, when union rapidly follows.

If a large dose of opium had been administered on the battle field, or as soon as the patient had arrived at the infirmary whilst awaiting his turn to be dressed, the peristaltic action of the bowels would have been suspended, and the wounded portion of the bowel, which should always be the last portion returned, when the hernia is extensive, remains within the abdominal cavity, in immediate contact with the wound, and to this point it soon becomes attached through adhesive inflammation. Should the sutures give way, or the bowel slough from the injury which it had received, its contents, instead of being thrown into the peritoneal cavity where it would produce fatal inflammation, on account of the adhesions of the bowel near an external outlet, will escape externally, which diminishes materially the risk run by the patient. The threads used in closing the opening in the intestine either escape through the bowel by stool, or are discharged through the abdominal wound.

When examining the external wound when no protrusion exist, should we find an escape of fecal matter—which proves that the bowel has been perforated—the abdominal wound must be enlarged, and the wound in the intestine closed by suture. This is the only expedient for saving life; for if the contents of the bowel are allowed to escape into the peritoneal cavity, a fatal issue must be expected. The dilatation of the wound diminishes the risks.

Should the intestine be extensively injured beyond the possibility of saving it, rather than return a portion of bowel within the abdomen to mortify and destroy the patient, it should be left hanging out of the wound. All of the sound portion of the protrusion having been returned, the crushed portion is enveloped in a wet or oiled cloth. The peritoneal coat of the bowel will form adhesions to the peritoneal edge of the abdominal wound, the outer portion sloughs, and an artificial anus gives constant escape to the fecal contents. In time, this artificial outlet gradually closes by a spontaneous effort of nature, the fæces seeking their normal passage, or an operation at some subsequent period removes the deformity.

In examining the archives of surgery, we find cases in which portions of the intestines have been cut off, the cylinder of the bowel reunited by sutures, and excellent recoveries obtained. These experiments have been tried successfully upon animals, and instances are met with where the human subject has been saved by a similar operation. I have recently had under my care a lunatic, who, some months since, attempted suicide by opening his abdomen, drawing out his bowels, and cutting off two feet of intestine. Dr. Gaston, of Columbia, S. C., who had the case under charge, brought the two ends of the intestine together, and securing them by carefully arranged sutures, returned them within the cavity. The patient made a perfect recovery. This accident, which terminated so successfully for the lunatic, suggests an operation for a crushed intestine, which may offer better prospects than leaving the bowel to slough and form an artificial anus:—remove the injured portion, secure the bleeding vessels, and reclose the intestine by sutures, treating the case as if an incised wound of the bowel had alone existed.

In all perforating wounds of the abdomen, as we cannot tell, in the absence of symptoms, whether the intestines have been injured or not, there are two fundamental rules of treatment never to be forgotten, and which are required in every instance.

1. Give opium freely and frequently, with a double object, viz: of controlling the peristaltic action, which alone can prevent extravasation of the contents into the peritoneal cavity, and for its antiphlogistic effect, to equalize the circulation, allay pain, suspend nervous irritability, and prevent inflammation.

2. Avoid the use of purgatives.

With the majority of physicians who have had but little experience in the treatment of abdominal wounds, the first impulse is to see the bowels emptied, and hence the fatal purgative is eagerly administered. An evacuation apparently reassures them that all is right; when on the contrary, all is very wrong, as the march of the case will soon show them. This is a fatal error, which the utmost after-care cannot remedy. For three or four days at least after the receipt of injury, in which the intestines are known or are supposed to be wounded, absolute rest, the most abstemious diet, and the liberal use of opium (one grain of gum opium, or its equivalent in laudanum, every five hours) in connection with cold water or iced dressing, will compose the entire treatment. If the patient feels uneasy, an enema will relieve the large intestines and add much to his comfort. By the fourth day, the wound in the intestines will have closed by lymphy effusion, and the dangers will, to a certain degree, have subsided. If required, a dose of Epsom salts, citrate of magnesia, or castor oil, may now be given, although it would be better to wait one or two days longer, when the risks of reopening or disturbing the wound would be but slight.

If peritoneal inflammation be excited with febrile reaction, with pain greatly increased by pressure over the abdomen, more particularly in the neighborhood of the wound, with tympanitis, vomiting, hiccup, small, quick pulse, and anxiety of countenance, the fears are that lymph and sero-purulent matter will be rapidly thrown out, gluing coils of intestines together, and filling the cavity with fluid. To check this rapidly fatal disorganization, leeches or cups should be applied to the abdomen, to be followed by ice bladders, which are now preferred, or by hot narcotic or turpentine stupes, or by blisters, whilst opium should be given in large doses and at short intervals. If the patient be young and plethoric, and the inflammatory symptoms are early recognized, the lancet might be used; but usually in military surgery this remedy is badly borne. Calomel was formerly used with the opium, and was considered the main dependence, but is now being generally discarded, as all advantages gained are accredited to the opium.

Sometimes, in a few hours, usually at the end of the second or third day, collapse, with a cold, sweating skin, and feeble, irregular pulse, shows the ravages which the system has experienced from the peritoneal inflammation, and marks rapidly-approaching dissolution. It is rare that the liberal use of brandy with carbonate of ammonia, external warmth and synapisms rescue the patient at this advanced stage; although, if given when debility commences to show itself, they may support the patient, and be the means of saving life. When the swelling of the abdomen, and the dull sound which percussion elicits, shows extensive effusion, the abdominal wound should be reopened, and, by placing the patient in a proper position, the effusion be allowed to escape. It is a desperate operation, but has been known to save a few cases, which, if left alone, would have certainly perished as those do upon whom this operation is not performed.

In gunshot wounds of the abdomen, if the missile has perforated, it would be madness to probe the abdominal cavity. We must imagine the worse, give the patient the benefit of these doubts, and by extreme care hope to counteract the baneful influences which foreign bodies, when remaining in the abdominal cavity, always exercise. The ball may have traversed the cavity and embedded itself in the fleshy walls without having injured any organ of importance in its course; the absence of serious symptoms, as the case progresses, can alone inform us on this head. From the physiological effects we might, at times, trace the resting place of the ball. When paralysis of the lower limbs follows an abdominal gunshot wound, we might infer the burying of the ball in the vertebral column, or an injury to the nerves of the extremity as they emerge from the spine, etc.

Should the abdominal wound bleed profusely, the source of blood may be from within the cavity from injured viscera, or may be caused by division of the epigastric artery in the abdominal walls. If the latter, dilatation of the wound will expose it, and the vessel should be ligated.

When from the former source but little can be done, venesection to syncope might check the flow, and the formation of a clot may plug up the injured vessel. Some surgeons, knowing the desperate condition brought on by internal hemorrhage, recommend dilating the wound, and should it be found that hemorrhage comes from one of the mesenteric vessels, the artery should be ligated. The position of the external wound will assist us in forming a diagnosis as to the probable source of the hemorrhage. Cases of recovery are recorded where the wound was dilated, and the bleeding vessel in the omentum sought and secured.

Where some of the large viscera or blood-vessels are injured in perforating abdominal wounds, the symptoms are much more marked than in intestinal wounds; hemorrhage at once takes place to a serious and often fatal extent. Such wounded are often found dead upon the battle field; or should they be alive, they are pale and cold, with anxious countenances and intense longing for water. This insatiable thirst is not peculiar to visceral wound or to nervous shock, but is an indication of serious hemorrhage. If the wound be extensive they never rally from this collapse. In other cases, the shock may permit the clogging of injured blood-vessels, and stop internal bleeding. Should life be prolonged until reaction takes place, the violent inflammation which is lit up, either from direct injury to the peritoneum, or from the quantity of blood in the cavity, usually carries off the patient after a period of intense suffering. On account of the hemorrhage and subsequent inflammation which accompany these injuries, all wounds of the larger abdominal viscera are considered nearly necessarily mortal, as the exceptional cures are very rare. When the external orifice is small, the position and direction of the wound will lead us to suspect the special injury, and, in connection with persistent vomiting, the ejection of blood by the mouth, by stool, or with the urine; the escape of special secretions, as bile, urine, or fæces by the wound; and the peculiar pain or sensations experienced by the patient, will be our chief indications in determining the part injured.

The treatment of these serious wounds, which on the whole is so unsatisfactory, is similar to that required for perforating wounds of the chest, with injury to the lungs. If seen soon after the accident, before much blood has been extravasated, and if nervous shock is not present, the patient should be bled nearly to syncope for its anti-hemorrhagic effect, and then opium internally, and cold locally, become the basis of treatment.

In wounds of the kidney, frequent micturition with bloody urine marks the injury; whilst in *injuries to the bladder*, bloody urine, or rather, the passage of clots as well as pure blood through the penis, is the diagnostic sign: should urine escape from the wound, it is equally pathognomonic. In addition to the course already laid down for internal abdominal injuries, the introduction of a large gum catheter into the bladder through the penis, through which urine is allowed to drain away as fast as it is secreted, will prevent urinous infiltration, which is one of the most fatal complications connected with a wounded bladder. The catheter should be introduced on the field of battle, and should be worn continuously for four or five days until adhesive inflammation has closed the torn cellular tissue, and shut up the avenues into which the urine would have escaped. The catheter will also be required when the sloughs are separating, as swelling of the parts often obstructs the ready flow of urine. The gum catheter may even be kept in from the commencement of the treatment until the wound is well advanced in healing, unless it excites much irritation, when it may be temporarily withdrawn. This precaution will prevent many cases of urinous infiltration and save many lives.

When the neck of the bladder, or the prostatic part of the urethra has been divided, if the catheter cannot be introduced, a free incision should be made through the perineum for the evacuation of urine and the discharges from the wound.

Injury to the large intestines are not so serious as perforations of the small. As the large bowel is bound down in the greater part of its course, extravasations of their contents do not necessarily take place into the peritoneal cavity; and although fecal matter escapes externally from the wound, and high inflammation, with profuse suppuration, usually follows, many of the wounded eventually do well.

Cases not unusually occur on the battle field in which the abdominal contents might be severely crushed without apparent external injury. It is the toughness and elasticity of the skin which gives rise to the exploded theory of the wind of a ball destroying life; and such cases as those we are now considering were formerly brought forward as instances of the fatal effects of the vacuum following the wake of a cannon ball. Observation has shown that a knapsack might be torn from the back, a hat struck from the head, an epaulet from the shoulder, or a pipe from the mouth, without leaving a trace of injury, whilst, on the other hand, viscera might be reduced to a jelly, or bones crushed, without visible bruising of the skin. It is the ball itself, and not the wind, which produces these disorganizations. From the blow of a spent cannon ball or fragment of shell, the liver might be lacerated, intestines torn, blood-vessels opened, spleen fissured, or kidney ruptured, without an external wound. Severe shock and collapse mark the extent of injury received; and should the patient rally from this condition, which is rare, violent inflammation will soon destroy life. Although we follow vigorously the treatment laid down above, we very seldom have the satisfaction of saving a patient.

The amount of destruction effected by a spent ball is often surprising. The uninitiated on the battle field will attempt to stop, with the foot, a cannon ball rolling on the ground, and which is just about exhausting its force, perhaps with only momentum sufficient to carry it one or two feet further, yet it crushes the limb put out to oppose it. Baudens, in warning persons to avoid cannon balls, however slowly they may be rolling on the ground, mentions the case of a grenadier of the guard, sleeping on his side on the ground, who was instantly killed by a spent cannon ball, the blow from which luxated the vertebral column. The ball came with so little momentum that it rolled itself up in the hood of the soldier's overcoat, where it was found. It was just about to stop when it struck. One or two feet further, and its entire force would have been exhausted.

CHAPTER XI.

Injuries of the extremities; compound fractures; difference of treatment in the upper and lower limbs; importance of an early examination and adoption of a course of treatment within twenty-four hours after the receipt of accident—Compound fractures of the arm from shot wounds, when not implicating joints, do not require amputation; should the blood-vessels and nerves be crushed with the bone, then amputation necessary—When gunshot fractures implicate joints, resection or amputation is the only means of saving life; how resections are to be performed; special resections of shoulder, elbow, wrist—Resections and amputations of the inferior extremity—Primary and consecutive amputation; when, and under what circumstances should amputations be performed—Modes of operating and of dressing stumps—Chloroform in all serious operations.

As the major portion of the injuries of the extremities are merely flesh wounds, these will not require to be again noticed. Those which we will now consider are such as involve the bones, joints, or important vessels, and which may call for special treatment. It is in this department that conservative surgery has made the greatest advances, and has accomplished so much in diminishing mortality and mutilation. Not that amputations will ever be abolished, for many lives can be saved in no other way than by the sacrifice of limbs; but conservative surgery has shown that the constant flourish of the amputating knife is not the way to obtain the greatest number of surgical victories in times of war. Amputations must, however, ever remain a surgical necessity; and he who removes crushed limbs with the greatest skill, and saves the patient by successful after-treatment, will ever deserve the high position which humanity and philanthropy will bestow upon him.

In gunshot wounds of the extremities, we find a much greater vitality and resistance to injuries in the upper than in the lower limbs, which would modify the treatment of similar injuries located in these two portions of the body. This depends upon the greater vascularity and freer anastomosis in the arm than in the leg. In the more liberal supply of blood-vessels and nerves, we find the source of safety which enables us to save an arm, when, for a similar injury, a leg would be generally condemned.

The most common accidents of the extremities which give surgeons the greatest annoyance and require the most careful diagnosis, prognosis and treatment, are *compound fractures.* These have always been a numerous and important class in military surgery, but have become doubly so in modern warfare, from the substitution of conical shot for the round musket ball. This projectile never impinges upon a bone without leaving frightful traces of devastation. Such a conical ball very rarely remains embedded, but acting on the principle of a wedge, it splits and comminutes the bone, driving the loose spiculæ in every direction, and even detaching some of them from the body to impale neighboring soldiers. Crimean surgeons, who have had many opportunities of observing injuries, from every description of missile, in referring to the conical ball, speak of their effects as so dissimilar to those of round balls, as almost to justify a classification of injuries founded upon the kind of ball giving rise to them. They state that the longitudinal splitting of the bone is so dexterously and extensively accomplished by the conical ball, that while only a small opening leads to the seat of fracture, the whole shaft may be rent from end to end. Fortunate is it that this extensive splitting or fissuring of the long bones does not extend into the joints, or the cases for operation would be much more numerous than they now are. The epiphysis of the bone appears not to transmit the force of cleavage, as the injury most frequently stops at the junction of the head of the bone with its shaft. The successful treatment of such wounds requires much judgment and experience, with a thorough knowledge of those agencies antagonistic to the healing of wounds, and which belong to military surgery.

When a bone is crushed by a ball, the patient is conveyed very carefully to the field infirmary; or, if it can be done without delay, to the general hospital, where the treatment commences. On the field, the ambulance surgeon can do nothing but administer a dose of morphine, and secure the limb to a rough splint to facilitate transportation. For a fractured clavicle, scapula or humerus, the arm is bandaged to the chest, which, on the battle field, answers the purpose of a temporary splint; for a crushing of the forearm or hand, the arm is laid upon a broad splint, and slung from the neck. If the splint is not at hand, the sling made of a handkerchief must answer until the wounded man can be better attended to; it being understood that a wet or greased cloth is always put over the wound for its protection during the transportation.

When he arrives at the hospital, the limb is carefully examined. The external wound may give no indication of the extent of internal injury. When the finger is introduced and the wound carefully explored, the degree of crushing will be ascertained, and the question at once proposes itself, what course shall we pursue? Shall we attempt to save the limb; or does its condition, with the want of proper facilities for its successful treatment, necessitate its condemnation? If we have had experience in the care of gunshot fractures, we should, with Sir Charles Bell, contemplate what will be the condition of the parts in twelve hours, in six days, or in three months. "In twelve hours the inflammation, pain and tension of the whole limb, the inflamed countenance, the brilliant eye, the sleepless and restless condition, declare the impression the injury is making on the limb and on the constitutional powers. In six days, the limb, from the groin to the toe, or from the shoulder to the finger, is swollen to half the size of the body; a violent phlegmonous inflammation pervades the whole; serous effusion has taken place in the whole limb, and abscesses are forming in the great beds of cellular texture throughout the whole extent of the extremity. In three months, if the patient has labored through the agony, the bones are carious; the abscesses are interminable sinuses; the limb is undermined and everywhere unsound, and the constitutional strength ebbs to the lowest degree." All these conditions must be rapidly considered, and with them the more immediate dangers of mortification, and the remote dangers of erysipelas, pyæmia and hectic, and the questionable utility of the limb, when, after several months of continued trials, the wound has been healed.

Business presses and time is valuable. Within twenty-four hours, or before reaction ensues, whilst the patient has his sensibilities depressed by the shock, our conclusions must be made and acted upon; success of treatment depends upon prompt action — the delay of a few days has destroyed thousands of wounded. Should amputation be required, there is no period in the progress of the case so favorable for the performance of this operation as the first four and twenty hours. Should an injudicious attempt be made to save the limb, amputation cannot be resorted to with any hope of success until suppurative action has been well established. Should erysipelas attack the wound, an amputation is impracticable; and when gangrene has supervened, during the stage of reactionary excitement, we are driven to an operation under the most unfavorable circumstances.

There are many compound fractures upon which judgment can be immediately passed: with some, there is every probability that the limb can be saved; whilst there are others in which the limb is condemned at a glance—our prognosis being based upon the following circumstances:

As the upper extremity can sustain a much more serious injury than the lower, we may lay it down as a rule that a simple compound fracture of any of the long bones of the arm, when not complicated with excessive crushing of the soft parts, can, and should be saved. An arm is rarely to be amputated except from the effects of a cannon shot, which, beside crushing the bones, makes frightful lacerations of the soft tissues, tearing away muscles, nerves, and blood-vessels, and often amputating completely the limb—the surgeon being required only to give a better form to the stump.

For a gunshot wound from a musket or Minnié

ball, which has fractured the bones of the arm without implicating a joint, the following is the course to be pursued. At the field infirmary the wound is carefully probed with the finger, and its spiculated condition noted. All loose fragments are to be removed at this first examination before reaction ensues, for it will be very injurious to the wound, as well as excessively painful to the soldier, to continue such examinations from day to day. The first examination should always be effectual. The patient is then suffering from shock, with sensibility temporarily blunted, and is therefore in the best condition to be operated upon. To render this first examination complete, should the shock have passed off and the patient complain of much pain, it would be better to give him large doses of opium, or administer chloroform, rather than desist from this important portion of the treatment. Should we omit to bring away all spiculæ, the further removal should not be attempted during the stage of excitement and febrile reaction which will come on after twenty-four hours, and which will run its course in six or eight days. When this subsides, then and not before, we make the second examination, and by the use of instruments, remove any loose fragments which we now detect. We will simply mention, in this connection, that as there is not the slightest probability, or even possibility, of the wound closing by the first intention, the insertion of tents and pieces of lint is a relic of barbarous surgery, which cannot be too severely condemned as useless, injurious, and very painful.

Modern surgery recommends that all spiculæ, whether detached or not, should be removed; but this practice is not upheld by surgeons generally. Experience and observation has, in some instances shown, that although the larger fragments may be detached from the shaft of the bone, they may still be adherent to the periosteum, which will effect a reunion and consolidation. On the other hand, experience and observation have shown that, from the force with which conical shot strike a bone, the spiculæ, which are very numerous, are driven in every direction, but mostly toward the opening of escape of the ball. These sharp splinters cannot but produce excessive irritation in the soft parts, and máy, by transfixing vessels, pricking nerves, or irritating muscles, induce hemorrhage, mortification, or tetanus. No surgeon doubts the propriety of removing all such on the spot, or at the earliest possible moment. As the opening of exit, around which the larger number of the fragments are found, may be too contracted to admit of a thorough exploration of the wound, it will not increase the dangers but, on the contrary, materially diminish the risks of after-trouble, if the wound of exit, in compound fractures with crushing of the bone, be dilated so as to facilitate the detection and removal of every spicula. In enlarging this orifice, injury to the important blood-vessels and nerves will, of course, be avoided.

On the subject of removing *all* fragments, whether detached or not, there appears to be a diversity of opinion, which is based upon the changes introduced into modern warfare. The older surgeons, who base their treatment on the effects of the musket ball, know that often the connection of the fragments to the soft parts and to the periosteum will guarantee a consolidation of the fragments. The round ball simply breaks the bone without scattering the fragments, and therefore their relations to the surrounding tissues will not be so materially changed. But notwithstanding this impression, which may or may not be correct, what does actual experience prove, when brought down to facts? Take the experience given by the inmates of the Hotel des Invalides, as recorded by M. Hutin, the surgeon of the institution. He states, that those spiculæ which had been attached to the soft parts, and which were allowed to remain in the hope of reunion, although they may not give trouble at the moment, invariably end by becoming sequestra, and after a long period of pain and suppuration, demand removal. He reports several hundred cases in which the non-extracted fragments, sooner or later, set up an eliminative action, which is always painful, often dangerous, and at times fatal. M. Hutin refers chiefly to the effects of round or musket balls. Baudens gives, as his Crimean experience, "that whether adherent or not, it is better to remove all spiculæ, and thus simplify the wound. If these be retained, endless suppuration, continued suffering, with exacerbations of all the symptoms at the escape of each fragment, will gradually exhaust the vital forces, and entail its sequelæ of marasmus, diarrhœa and hectic." Suppuration will eventually bring all of the fragments to the surface, but at what a sacrifice!

McLeod, after quoting the experience of Roux, Baudens, Guthrie, Hutin, Dupuytren, Curling, Begin, and others, on the dangers of allowing movable fragments to remain, and the necessity of extracting every piece which is not extensively attached to the soft parts, gives his experience as decidedly in favor of the modern practice of removing *all movable spiculæ* as the best mode of hastening a cure and diminishing mortality, "as the removal must tend immensely to simplify the wound."

Again, he says: "The extensive comminution of the bone by a conical ball, makes the indications with regard to the management of the sequestra more evident than it is commonly considered. I do not think that we paid sufficient attention to their removal in the East. It may be true, as some tell us, that in fractures with the old ball, it was desirable to meddle as little as possible with the fragments; but this is the teaching of only a few. However, to my mind, the question assumes a totally different light when viewed by the pathological results which we had occasion to witness."

Some surgeons go further, and recommend that not only should all spiculæ be removed, but that the sharp, irregular ends of the bones should be sawed off. This suggestion has not met with general approval, and is spoken of by Stromyer and Loeffler as no improvement. Their experience gave a larger mortuary list when this practice was attempted.

There is no doubt that the removal of all fragments, in which there is not a strong probability of reunion taking place, will expedite the cure. In surgery, whenever we are in doubt, we should always give the patient the benefit of it; and in the subject under consideration, knowing that the removal of spiculæ, which might effect consolidation, can do no harm, whilst leaving them in, should union not be obtained, would be followed by much danger, annoyance, and suffering, we give the patient the benefit of the doubt, and remove them at the first examination. Feeling now secure, that we have removed every foreign body, and have left nothing in the wound which is likely to retard the cure, we should ignore the presence of the wound as much as possible, and treat the case as one of simple fracture. Inflammation and suppuration we expect; they are the portion of compound fractures generally, and especially of those connected with gunshot wounds; and remembering the long continued and profuse drain which will establish itself in four or five days, we should be careful how we make use of the active antiphlogistic treatment. For the first week or ten days, the arm may be stretched upon a pillow, or loosely secured to a broad, long splint, which will support the entire extremity. We confine the treatment to cold water dressings, either as iced bladders, applied over compresses to remove the injurious effects of direct application, or as by the process of irrigation—either of which is better than the continued renewal of wet cloths. The general treatment during this period of inflammatory excitement, is diet, rest, quiet, and the use of mild diaphoretics, diuretics, and the liberal use of opium.

Pain we do not consider, in any sense, necessary to the healing of wounds, and therefore have always made it a rule in practice to reduce it to its minimum. The complete annihilation of pain will neither detract from the rapidity of healing, nor from the gratitude of patients. The impropriety of free catharsis, will be at once evident from the movements made necessary by their action. Bloodletting, emetics, and the use of mercury we absolutely discard, as always useless and injurious in the treatment of any stage of compound fractures. As soon as the period of inflammatory reaction has subsided, we then apply such splints to the arm as will secure quiet and rest to the limb, whilst a free vent is allowed in the apparatus for the escape of discharges from the wound; this opening also permits water dressings being applied to the wound.

It cannot be expected that an arm, after a serious gunshot injury to the bones, will be cured without deformity. The arm will always be shortened, where many spiculæ have been removed. We acknowledge this fact in anticipation, and never attempt, by traction and counter-extension, to restore it to its former length. We simply place the arm in an easy position and allow the muscles to approach the broken ends. In the treatment of ordinary fractures, the main object is to prevent deformity, and especially shortening of the limb. As this object is discarded in compound fractures of the upper extremity, the treatment becomes much simplified, and the patient is saved its greatest annoyance.

In fractures of the arm, the pasteboard splints are to be preferred; whilst for the forearm, wooden splints, made of light material and wider than the diameter of the arm, will make the best application. The tumefaction bandage is not now insisted on, and by many surgeons is nearly altogether discarded. In gunshot injuries, where we have an open wound to dress daily, our mechanical applications should be of such a character as to permit of easy inspection and also the ready re-adjustment of the apparatus when disarranged; whilst, at the same time, the splints are kept secure. Diachylon plaster is now extensively used to secure splints to fractured limbs: three or four bands encircling the limb will always secure the supporting apparatus, whilst the limb is freely open to inspection. When the pasteboard is moistened, it moulds itself to the arm and makes a very satisfactory dressing.

As soon as the patient has passed the reactive stage, he should no longer be confined to his bed, but with his arm in a sling may obtain sufficient exercise to keep his system in good order. The erect position will have the additional advantage of permitting the ready discharge of pus, and will prevent the bagging of this fluid, and obviate the necessity for the establishment of counter-openings. In all simple fractures the excess of callus depends upon the degree of mobility between the broken ends; in compound fractures the deposit for consolidation is usually very great, which may be explained by the amount of irritation from inflammatory action, and also by the difficulty of keeping the fragments without motion. Fortunately, this does not interfere with the final results, as false joints are not more frequently met with in compound than in simple fractures. Experience shows us that there is not that necessity, which many practice, of frequently tightening the apparatus, to the very great annoyance of the patient. If the constitution be strong, a considerable degree of relaxation may be permitted, and be found not incompatible with perfect consolidation. In animals with compound fractures, we see continual exemplifications of this fact.

The local and general treatment of the wound, will, in no respect, be modified on account of the fracture. Water dressings, until cicatrization is completed, medicated with astringents to allay profuse discharges, or with antiseptics to remove fœtor, or with stimuli to promote granulations, will be the proper course, whilst the general health is watched, retarded secretions promoted, and debility guarded against. If any fragments of bone have been left in, and have become necrosed, the surgeon must assist nature in the expulsion as soon as they have become detached, otherwise they will become surrounded by new formations, and as sequestra, incarcerated in an involucrum, will only be expelled after much time and trouble. From time to time, when spiculæ are suspected, the wound should be examined, especially about the eighth or tenth day from the receipt of injury, when the stage of reaction has subsided to such an extent that the finger can again be introduced. From the passing off of the shock, all examination must be absolutely interdicted until the period of reaction has subsided. During the first week, no one should be permitted to probe the wound. As soon as we conclude that all fragments have been removed, we desist from all further probing, as it cannot but be injurious to the delicate granulations.

Cleanliness is necessary to successful hospital practice in the treatment of suppurating wounds, but, when excessive, becomes a serious obstacle to rapid cicatrization. It is a common error for surgeons to place a wounded limb over a basin of water, and sponge and rub it as if they were cleansing a piece of porcelain. I have seen others dress gunshot wounds by the free use of a powerful syringe, with which they poured a stream of water into the wound until the granulations were bleached, and this repeated with great regularity at the morning and evening visit. It was not surprising that wounds, treated with this over-care, took a very long time to heal. If the wound be gangrenous, and the object be to remove ichorous decomposing fluids, to diminish or prevent absorption and general poisoning, then the syringing is desirable; but under no other conditions wipe or wash the granulating surface of a wound. Wipe around the edges and remove any secretions which might have collected upon the skin, but leave the pus, as the best covering which healthy granulations can have. Under its protection, the plasma, which is thrown out from the blood-vessels, will rapidly form tissues; but rub or wash away this covering, and the exposure to the baneful influences of the atmosphere will rapidly destroy the granulations which had already formed. However useful the local and general bath is to advance the cicatrization of a suppurating wound, do not generalize too much and expect equally good service from cleansing the granulations.

Compound fractures, under the very best conditions, are tedious cases, and in gunshot injuries our patience will often be taxed to the utmost. Despondency should not be an element in the character of a military surgeon. We must expect to have a compound fracture under treatment at least twice, if not three times as long as would be required to consolidate a simple fracture.

Should the main vessel be injured, in connection with the fractured bones, we still have not sufficient cause to sacrifice the limb; but, ligating the artery at its bleeding mouths, we treat the fracture as if this complication had not existed. Owing to the free anastomosis of the blood-vessels of the arm, mortification is not to be feared when a ligation is applied even to the brachial artery; a circuitous route soon supplies the needful nourishment to the parts beyond. Should the nerves as well as the artery be injured, or the principal nerves alone with the bones, then the limb, even when saved, would be a useless, paralyzed extremity, and its immediate removal will save the patient a long, tedious, and dangerous convalescence. In such cases, it is our duty to sacrifice the limb to diminish the risks to life.

The most dangerous fractures of the extremities are those involving the heads of the bones and extending into a joint. The synovial injury adds greatly to the danger of the case, and in former times was considered nearly a fatal complication, as it necessitated an amputation, which, under the ordinary circumstances attending hospital treatment, was not far removed from an early dissolution. Nor have we much to boast of: for, when amputations near the trunk are required, notwithstanding all the improvements in modern science, we succeed but little better in checking the fearful mortality. The severity of the symptoms of articular injuries depend upon the size of the joint and the character of the wound. The dangers are serious enough with the smallest puncture, but when the wound is large and lacerated, extensive local mischief and constitutional disturbance is sure to ensue, leading with certainty to the destruction of the joint, and usually destroying the patient. Hence, in the days of John Bell, the united experience of surgeons considered wounds of joints mortal. Crimean experience corroborates John Bell's conclusions, as no serious injury to the large joints recovered unless the limbs were amputated or joints resected. The great fear is not in the serious injuries, as these cases are at once operated upon. It is in the apparently trivial cases, where, from the very small size of the wound, we hope that no trouble will supervene, that violent inflammation shows itself and life is sacrificed.

A wounded joint, under the ordinary hospital treatment, will pursue the following course:

When a ball has perforated the joint, the period of reaction is not long absent. In extensive wounds a great degree of nervous shock accompanies the injury, the patient lying deadly pale, cold and faint. In from twelve to twenty-four hours, the tissues around the articulation become hot, swollen, and painful; inflammation has already seized upon the synovial membrane, and will soon involve all the structures. All the symptoms rapidly increase until they become excessive. There is no rest for the weary sufferer, who, in spite of iced applications, and the free use of morphine, with the entire arcana of antiphlogistic remedies, writhes about in unmitigated agony. If the aperture leading into the joint be made by a ball or piece of shell, the synovia at first, and in two or three days pus freely escapes. Should the entrance into the joint be small or the passage oblique, the purulent synovia fills and distends the joint, adding much to the agony, which is again increased by the irregular spasmodic contractions of the surrounding muscles. Accompanying these local symptoms will be found a high grade of inflammatory fever, with rigors determined, great gastric distress, intense thirst, excessive restlessness, and with such an amount of constitutional disturbance as sometimes to destroy life in a few days. As the disease advances, abscesses form in the surrounding tissues by extension of the inflammatory process, and in a few days open continuous passages to the joint, from which a constant discharge of purulent matter escapes. If the patient is not destroyed in the early stages of the disease by erysipelas, pyæmia, etc., in connection with the irritative fever, he falls a prey to hectic, caused by the continued drain from the disorganized joint; synovial membrane, cartilages, and bones forming one mass of disease. In gunshot wounds of joints, very rarely does the patient escape with life in military hospitals. In private practice he sometimes recovers, but even under the most advantageous circumstances a successful case is rarely seen, and then usually with a destroyed anchylosed joint. As the results in injured joints are so fatal, surgeons had, at an early day, adopted amputations as giving the only chance for recovery. In recent years, conservative surgery has introduced the operation of resection as affording not only the means of preserving life, but also of saving a useful limb.

The diagnosis of articular injury is usually evident from the direction of the wound, and from the escape of synovia; at times, however, when the orifice is small and the wound circuitous, a successful diagnosis requires much experience and close observation. When possible, a consultation should always be had over these cases. It is in these very cases of doubt, or of apparently trivial injury, that the most violent reactionary symptoms are met, and that a fatal issue occurs. If left unoperated upon, the trifling wound, perforating the joint, might nearly be considered mortal; whilst, if the joint be not implicated, the operation of resection is not only not called for, but unnecessarily risks the life of the individual. The urgent necessity for an accurate diagnosis is evident.

For the upper extremity this resource is particularly applicable, as resection is now the rule of practice, having superseded amputation in all cases where the blood-vessels and nerves around the joint are not involved in the injury. When a joint has in any way been injured by a gun-shot wound, whether the articulation has only been opened, or the heads of the bones forming it crushed, as soon as the excessive shock under which the patient may be suffering passes off, we proceed at once to operate. A primary resection is as essential as a primary amputation, and is followed by as successful results. It should be performed within twenty-four or thirty-six hours, or before reaction sets in. Such cases do much better could the patient have been transferred to the general hospital prior to an operation, as transportation is difficult and dangerous immediately after the resection, from the difficulty of securing the limb from movements. Should the case not come under observation until reaction has come on, then by general, mild, antiphlogistic treatment, and ice bladders or cold water dressings locally, we await the establishment of suppuration, when the operation might be attempted with good prospects of success.

The results of the primary resection are more successful than the secondary; and these are, in turn, much more likely to succeed than when the operation is performed during the stage of febrile excitement. There are three or four rules necessary in all cases of resection, and which should not be forgotten during the operation, viz: Make the incision for exposing the heads of the bones in that portion of the extremity opposite to the main blood-vessels and nerves, so that these may not be exposed to injury. If possible, make the wound lie in the line of the incision, and place the incisions in such a way as to permit a continued drain from the joint. Make these incisions free, so as not to cramp the operator in turning out the heads of the bones. An inch added to the incision does not increase its serious character, and hastens the operation. Remove most of the synovial membrane, and save as much periosteum as possible; the one is prone to take on inflammation; the other makes, and will, to a certain extent, reproduce the bone. In performing secondary resections, the removal of all the diseased synovial membrane becomes one of the first elements of success. More successes are obtained from resections of the shoulder joint than from any other articulation, the statistical tables of the final results of operations in favor of resection being conclusive over amputations.

The following is the course recommended for performing the operation of resection, a substitute for amputation of the arm:—a U shaped flap, about three inches in length, is made of the deltoid muscle, on the upper and outer portion of the arm; if there be any wound on this portion of the extremity, making one arm of the incision include the wound. The knife passing directly to the bone, from the clavicle or accromial process downward for three inches, makes a large flap of the deltoid, which is raised by a few touches of the knife. The circumflex arteries are divided in this first incision, and should be at once ligated, otherwise, as they are of considerable size, the patient will lose much blood, and the steps of the operation obscured. By carrying the arm over the chest, the capsule of the joint is exposed and divided transversely, and with it the rotary muscles of the shoulder, when the head will protrude from its position. The long head of the biceps is carefully removed from its bicepital groove and protected from injury. The bones are now examined; a knife blade, or spatula, as a guard, is placed behind the bone so as to protect the soft parts and vessels from injury, and all of the injured portion is removed. When the ball has entered directly within the joint, only the surface may require excision; but should the head of the bone be extensively spiculated, we must cut back to the sound bone, even if we are compelled to remove four or five inches of the shaft of the bone, as was successfully done by Stromyer for a gunshot injury: should the glenoid cavity be equally injured, the fractured portion is removed. The rule is, never to remove more of the bone than is absolutely called for, and not to open the medullary cavity if it can in any way be avoided.

When the wound has been cleansed of all foreign bodies, the flap is replaced and secured with one or two points of suture. As adhesion by the first intention is not usually expected, and gives no advantage over the final result by granulation, nice adjustment is not necessary. The patient is then put to bed and cold water dressings applied. Inflammation at first runs high, the parts around the joint are much swollen, and a collection soon forms within the cavity from which the bones have been removed. The escape of this decomposed blood and pus from the wound gives great relief. When kept in by the too nice adjustment of the flap, the collection increases the swelling, œdema, and pain which it diffuses over the neighboring parts, involving the chest as well as arm. When suppuration becomes established, the swelling and pain subside; granulations spring up, and eventually close the wound. In the meantime the divided muscles have formed new relations by a lymphy exudation; they become more or less incorporated with the surrounding tissues, and by taking an insertion around the cut portion of the bone, form in time a closed capsule. A head to the bone is sometimes, in a measure, formed; in other cases the head of the bone becomes attached to the cavity by fibrinous bands. Of the cases of resection of the shoulder performed in the Crimea but few died; and all those saved regained a useful limb, possessing all the motions, with the exception of those of the deltoid, which muscle is, to a certain extent, paralyzed from the division of its nerves, which cannot altogether be avoided in exposing the head of the bone.

As suppuration will be excessive, and often long-continued, nourishment and even stimuli may be demanded during the treatment. When abscesses form in the surrounding cellular tissue they should be open. It is a matter of but little importance in what position the limb is placed, and how it is secured, provided its position is comfortable to the sufferer. The uneasiness and irritation which the splints and bandages give, do much to prevent success. It matters little what length of limb the patient has, provided his life be saved, and the convalescence be speedy. A shortened arm does not affect its usefulness, and a slightly changed direction can be corrected in the after-stages of the treatment. The most effectual management is the simplest, and tedious daily dressings are to be discouraged; straightening the limb upon the bed, a pillow, or a long, broad splint, without bandaging, being the best and most comfortable dressing for any resection. The patient is kept in bed until the suppurative stage is established, when he will be permitted to get up. His arm is then placed in a sling, and the water dressings are continued until a complete cure is effected. When the parts are nearly cicatrized, it will be time enough to apply the tumefaction bandage, for removing the œdema of the limb. Anchylosis rarely follows this operation in the shoulder-joint. As a proof of the efficacy of resection, Stromyer excised nineteen shoulder-joints with a loss of seven, chiefly from pyæmia. Of eight cases in which the operation was required, but from some mitigating circumstances was not performed, five died.

Gunshot wounds in the neighborhood of the elbow-joint are much more readily recognized by the escape of the synovia, etc., than injuries of the shoulder. Inflammatory reaction runs high, as in all cases in which the joints have been opened by a ball. Collections soon form, and the excessive swelling stretches the softened capsule, which, giving way, allows of the burrowing of pus and final discharge through open abscesses. After running a tedious, painful, and dangerous course, if the patient escapes with a shattered constitution and an anchylosed limb, he is fortunate. A primary resection offers a diminution of the risks to life, a rapid convalescence, and a movable joint. In the Schleswig-Holstein army, of fifty-four amputations of the arm nineteen died, whilst of forty resections under similar circumstances only six died. The results of the operations were also modified by the period of performing the resection. Of eleven cases excised within twenty-four hours before reaction ensued, but one died; of twenty cases between the second and fourth day, or during the stage of irritation or excitement, four died; and of nine cases operated upon between the eighth and thirty-seventh day, only one died: an exemplification of a general rule laid down in the commencement of this chapter, that the wounded bear operations before the stage of reaction, or after the establishment of suppuration, much better than they do whilst suffering under high inflammatory excitement. This shows the necessity of deferring operations.

The elbow-joint, for gunshot wounds, transfixing its capsule and fracturing the bones, is best resected from the back of the joint, the patient lying upon his abdomen. An H, L, or T incision, taking in the breadth of the articulation, when sufficiently long, will expose perfectly the heads of the bones. There are no important vessels on this posterior portion of the arm, and only one nerve, the ulna, which must be sought on the inner side and avoided in the incision, or paralysis of all the muscles supplied by it will follow its section. When the posterior ligaments are divided, and the joint exposed, only remove the fractured head and all foreign bodies, and do not interfere with that bone which has not been injured. The lips of the wound are closed by sutures, and cold water dressings become the principal treatment. The limb is placed upon pillows, and not disturbed, if possible, until suppuration is established. When the soft parts are cicatrizing, and healing is nearly completed, passive motions in the joint will prevent anchylosis, and a tumefaction bandage will remove the œdema of the limb. Instances of good results are recorded for injuries at the wrist-joint, where the spiculated ends of both radius and ulna have been satisfactorily removed; also, instances in which either of these bones have been removed entire, for chronic ostitis and necrosis brought on from gunshot injuries. Similar incisions to those recommended for the resection of the elbow-joint will expose the heads of the wrist-bones, and permit of the ready removal of any injured portion. In this as in all other cases, we must save all tendons passing over a joint to supply distant bones; and in the wrist particularly, many of the muscles which supply the fingers can be drawn out of the way and thus escape injury.

However frightful an injury involves the hand, it is very seldom that it is so mangled as to be beyond the pale of surgical skill, and unless it is literally ground up it should not be amputated. In certain cases, fingers may have been already torn off, or may be hanging by a fragment of skin, when they should be removed; but for ordinary gunshot lacerations of the hand, amputation of the entire hand is very rarely required. Different bones of the hand and wrist are to be removed when irrevocably injured, with or without the metacarpal bones of the fingers or the thumb. Any fingers which can be saved will be better than the best artificial limb. In cases of lacerated hands in military surgery, when attempts are made to save the limb, under cold water dressings, the inflammation which comes on makes a shocking limb to those unaccustomed to treat lacerations of this extremity; but at the end of eight or ten days, when suppuration has been well established and granulations are forming, the swelling subsides, the torn portions are drawn together, cicatrization advances rapidly, and often but little deformity remains: at least the patient retains a useful limb. Some surgeons lay down the rule, that an amputation of the hand is never imperative, however frightful the injury to it may appear; and there is much truth in the assertion.

In the inferior extremity, we find the treatment of gunshot injuries somewhat different from those of the upper limb, on account of the minor degree of vascularity, and the much greater tendency to mortification, so that the rule to which we called attention, of amputations being rarely required for the superior extremity, is reversed for the leg, where it is often the only way of escape left to save the life of the wounded.

We have elsewhere stated that when balls embed themselves in the pelvic bones, and their position can be discovered, provided a serious operation is not needed, they should be removed, as their presence will, sooner or later, give rise to trouble; and also that all loose spiculæ should be taken away. Sequestra frequently show themselves from time to time during the treatment, and are withdrawn. When the ball strikes lower down, in the neighborhood of the trochanters, it usually splinters the bone, and frequently involves the ilio-femoral articulation. Such injuries are of the most serious character, and are usually considered fatal. It is a question of much moment to inquire, how can modern surgery, with all of its appliances, improvements and experience, assist in saving the life and limb of such seriously wounded? Within a few years the rule for all compound fractures of the femur was amputation of the limb; but the statistics from military hospitals in time of war are so frightful—but few successes for the numbers treated—that it was naturally suggested that the risks could not be materially increased by letting the patient take the chances with his limb on; when, if his life was saved, it would be with, and not without his leg. This has settled down into a conviction for fractures of the upper third of the femur, which are now treated without amputation, inasmuch as nearly every amputation in the neighborhood of the trochanter and all at the hip-joint are fatal. If we are assured that the ball has crushed the head of the bone, then the operation of resection offers the best prospects of success for the patient; but it does not always follow that this diagnosis can be clearly made out, if the signs of intra-capsular fracture be not present. Military surgical experience shows, that a fracture of the upper portion of the shaft of a bone does not necessarily extend into the head, and *vice versa*. Unless the junction of the epiphysis with the shaft is struck, the fracture is more apt to be confined to a centre of ossification, so that, in the thigh as in the arm, a blow just below the trochanter will not usually fracture the head of the femur. When the joint is opened and the head of the bone fractured, the wound should be enlarged, or an opening made into the joint from the outer side of the hip, by which the fractured head might be removed. If any success is hoped for, those cases alone should be selected in which neither blood-vessels nor nerves are injured, nor the soft parts extensively torn. If all or any of such are injured, where experience teaches us that the chances from successful resection are more than doubtful, do not have recourse to amputation which is so certainly fatal, but let the patient live his few remaining hours or days without being haunted by the ghost of a useless operation. Should he revive the reactionary stage, and still retain a good pulse and comparatively unshattered constitution, then a secondary operation might give a chance of success. In the Crimean service, no amputation in the vicinity of the hip-joint was successful—every individual case died. This only corroborates the experience of other campaigns, and shows the inutility of such mutilations. When death, from a crushed thigh-joint is inevitable, it is hardly humane to amputate under the plea of giving the patient the benefit of the chances which experience teaches us are nugatory.

As regards resections in suitable cases, the report is a little more satisfactory. Of six resections performed by the English surgeons in the

Crimea, one was successful, and the condition of all operated upon was made more comfortable. Had the conveniences for treatment been greater, and the general sanitary condition of the troops better, with less pyæmia, hospital gangrene and scurvy, much better results might have been obtained. Some of the cases were doing well, with every prospect of final success, when they were swept off by one of the above diseases. In amputations at the hip-joint, all the cases died speedily.

In cases of resection, the greatest difficulty lies in the after-treatment. As it is not expected to restore a perfect limb, no good result can be obtained by using violent extension. The leg, however, must be fixed, to facilitate those movements, in changing position, which are necessary to the patient's comfort. A long, straight splint is used for this purpose by some surgeons, whilst the incline-plane, which I would much prefer, is depended upon by others. Some have bandaged the limb to the sound one, and speak of it as a good mode of support. Water dressings compose the local treatment.

Baudens succeeded in saving both limb and life in cases in which compound fractures of the upper half of the thigh were treated without operation. Consolidated and useful limbs, with but little deformity, are reported as having been saved. By the use of the fracture box and incline-plane, he succeeded in curing a compound fracture on a level with the trochanter, saving a useful limb, although he had extracted two inches of the shaft of the femur. His experience proves that compound comminuted fractures of the upper half of the thigh are not so fatal when attempts are made to save the limb as when the thigh is amputated.

As the resection of the hip is so much more successful when performed for disease than for injury, it has been suggested by surgeons of experience, that an exception to the rule of immediate resections be made for the hip-joint, and that such cases, even the most suitable for the operation, be deferred until suppuration be well established. For hip-joint resections, it is said that nothing is lost by this delay, whilst, on the contrary, there may be a chance of saving the limb without an operation. Larrey, in 1812, reported six cases of gunshot fractures of the neck of the femur, with three cures, showing that the prospects are not altogether hopeless. When the patient is in a measure placed in similar conditions to those affected with diseases of the bones, his prospect for a successful resection appears to be improved. Baudens says, that as the resection of the hip-joint only succeeds as a secondary operation, attempts should first be made to save the limb.

We preface the following table, taken from Armand's Histoire Medico-Chirurgicale de la Guerre de Crimée, with the suggestion that any surgeon who has ever had a successful case of resection at the hip-joint, has always been eager to publish it; whilst many have been disposed to hide their misfortunes from the public, so that the tables, showing the relative advantages of primary and secondary resections, appear in their very best light.

PRIMARY RESECTIONS AFTER GUNSHOT WOUNDS.

SURGEONS:	Operated upon.	Cures.	Deaths.
Larrey. (Volume 3, Clinique)	6	..	6
J. Cooper. (Dictionary)	2	..	2
Leteille. (Relatione du Siege d'Anvers, par M. H. Larrey)	1	..	1
Hutin. (Memoires de Medicine et de Chirurgie Militaires)	2	..	2
Sedillot. (Annales de la Chirurgie Francaise et Étrangère)	5	..	5
Guyon. (Expédition de Churchill, Algérie)	1	..	1
Ruchet. (Journées de Juin, 1848)	1	..	1
Oubiot. (Thèse de Montpellier, 1840)	3	..	3
French Crimean Service	9	..	9
McLeod. (Crimean War)	5	1*	4
Stromyer	1	..	1
	36	1	35

* This successful case was found, after the articulation had been laid open, not to be a fracture extending within the joint, but confined without the capsule; and we are, therefore, justified in the belief that the case would have done equally well without the resection.

SECONDARY OPERATIONS FROM GUNSHOT WOUNDS.

Larrey. (Clinique, volume 5)............	1	1	..
Guthrie. (Clinic, volume 5).............	1	1	..
Baudens. (Traité des Plaies d'Armes a feu)	1	1	..
Ferussac. (Bulletin des Science Medicales, volume 3)...........................	1	..	1
Robert. (Journée de Juin, 1848).........	1	..	1
Guersant. (Journées de Juin, 1848)......	1	..	1
Vidal. (Traite de Chirurgie)............	1	..	1
Mounier. (Constantinople, 1854).........	3	..	3
Legouest. (Constantinople, 1854)........	1	..	1
McLeod. (Crimean War)...................	1	..	1
	12	3	9

It has been suggested, that if the patient who has been operated upon could have facilities for slinging the whole body, it would afford many advantages in the management of excisions of the hip-joint.

A compound fracture in the upper third of the thigh should be treated in every respect as if in the arm. Unless the leg is so mangled that an amputation is an act of necessity, it should not be thought of. We have already said that, in field military surgery, amputation near the trunk is synonymous with death. The treatment must commence on the battle field by proper transportation; as the judicious removal of fractured limbs is as important as an operation, and any neglect in this department will deprive the wounded man of all hope of retaining his limb, or often of having his life saved. We will carefully remove all loose and movable spiculæ, dilating the wounds if necessary, to facilitate the thorough cleansing of all foreign bodies. Until suppuration is well established, the limb is kept in an easy position and surrounded with cold applications. All tight, retentive bandages are to be rejected, as they interfere with topical antiphlogistic applications. Dispense with bandages. On the eighth or tenth day, when the reactionary stage has passed, the wound is again to be examined for foreign bodies, and all portions of bone which may have become separated by the inflammatory process must be removed; or as sequestra, they will become incorporated in the new osseous formations, and be the cause of much trouble and suffering.

In all compound fractures, with much loss of bone, it is always injurious to attempt to obtain a limb of equal length with the sound one. It cannot be done, and the chafing and annoyance of splints and tight bandaging may react very seriously, if not fatally upon the constitution. The first thing to be attended to is the facilities for treating such a fracture. If we are striving for successful results, we must not expect to obtain them if a patient, with a compound fracture of the thigh, is being treated upon the ground or is lying upon a little straw. He must have a proper bed and a good firm mattress, prepared with a bed-pan hole, for facilitating nature's daily wants without the necessity of moving him. Upon this the patient is placed, lying on his back, with the leg extended. Two long straps of diachylon plaster are attached to the sides of his leg from the knee to the ankle; they form a loop under the foot, and a weight is swung from this over the foot of the bed. This will be sufficient to tire the muscles and make the necessary degree of extension; or the limb might be loosely attached to a long thigh splint. The tumefaction roller is inadmissible, and strips of adhesive plaster, or strips of bandage, will secure the limb to the splint, and at the same time leave the wound open for inspection and dressing. For the first week or ten days this will be all the apparatus needed. As the case advances, splints may be more methodically applied by using long inner and outer splints of light board, well padded with loose cotton, and secured in position by bands of adhesive plaster or with tapes. The counter-extending bands are made by adhesive strips attached to the sides of the leg and carried under the foot, where they are secured to the end of the splint. Allow the ends of the bones to fill up the void made by the extraction of the spiculæ, as this hastens consolidation. With the exception of the mechanical appliances for the broken bone, the case is treated as for a long-continuous suppurating wound, by avoiding, in all cases, depletion and by giving liberal diet. Many of these cases will die; but if we have facilities in a well-ventilated and well-organized hospital, we will have the satisfaction of saving some of the patients submitted to our care.

In fractures of the middle and lower third of the thigh, not implicating the knee-joint, the question will again occur—what course is to be pursued with them? These are still very serious cases, and are classed with those of the upper third. Where attempts are made to save them, as recommended by Guthrie, the fatality will not be very dissimilar to fractures nearer the trunk, and the moderate success which, under the very best circumstances, we will obtain, will depend upon the state of health of the sufferer and the conveniences for treatment.

There are cases which often appear so trivial—only a small bullet hole leading to the crushed bone—that it seems barbarous surgery to condemn the limb without an attempt at saving it. The young military surgeon expects much from conservative surgery in such cases. We are informed by the experienced, that this striving after conservatism is the main cause of the heavy mortality. Surgeons generally are not prepared to believe how hopeless compound fractures of the thigh are, until the unwelcomed truth is forced upon them by an ever-recurring experience, that many lives are sacrificed to attempts at saving these broken limbs. In civil surgery, or with every facility in military hospitals, we should attempt to save the limb—it is the proper course to pursue; but on the battle field, with the deteriorated material upon which we are operating, and the poisoned atmosphere of the wards into which the patient is to be carried, it is a fatal error. Military surgeons must abandon their conservative intentions to expediency. It is for such cases that primary amputation offers the best chances for life. In rejecting amputations we lose more lives than we save limbs. As a rule, amputations are less hazardous the greater distance we operate from the trunk, and the reason why amputations are urged for compound fractures of the lower and not upper portions of the femur is, that the chances being similar without it, amputations are much less fatal in the lower than in the upper half of the thigh.

Resection of the shaft of the femur for a crushing of the bone has been often recommended and as often practiced, but the experience of latter years discourages its performance, as the operation is more serious than the condition for which the remedy is used. When the splinters of bone are removed, there is considerable space for the play of the rough edges remaining, and which, therefore, give but little trouble.

Should we attempt to save a fractured thigh in its lower third, we may use either the straight splint or the double incline-plane. The latter is much the more comfortable position for the patient, but has the disadvantage of promoting the burrowing of pus, which, in working its way down the limb, may dissect passages for itself as far as the buttock, and, by its multiplied openings, cause much annoyance as well as much destruction to bones and muscles. Surgeons in the Crimea often had cause to regret attempts at saving fractured thighs, but never regretted an early amputation.

When the knee-joint is implicated in a shot wound, or cut open by a shell, with injury to the head of the tibia or femur, experience has shown that, however trivial the wound may appear, if the synovial sac be entered, and air be admitted, or a foreign body lie within the joint, violent synovitis, with great pain, swelling and heat, and with excessive inflammatory fever, will come on after twenty-four or thirty-six hours. Should the patient survive the inflammatory stage, erysipelas, pyæmia or hectic will ultimately destroy life; and although on the other hand, the effusions may be absorbed, and a good anchylosed limb saved, it is a very rare occurrence. If the soft parts are not much lacerated, or the blood-vessels and nerves behind the joint injured, such cases are well adapted for resection, and excellent results are obtained in practice.

A straight or elliptical incision over the anterior portion of the joint, across its entire diameter, will expose the interior, and enable the surgeon to remove the foreign bodies, whatever they may be, and with them the head of the injured bones. The section of the bones should be made in such a way that the surfaces will adapt themselves to each other. When the external wound is closed by sutures, union by the first intention may, to a certain extent, be obtained. In the successful cases, the bones eventually become firmly united, and, with an anchylosed joint, the patient retains a useful limb. After the resection, a long splint upon the back of the leg, reaching from the buttock to the heel, is all the apparatus required, whilst cold water dressings are alone applied around the joint. In cases of resection, the surgeon must not expect quick union in the wound, as that does not often occur in military surgery. A tedious suppuration, the formation of numerous abscesses, and often the exfoliation of portions of bone is the rule, requiring care and judicious management to obtain a final success; many of those operated upon being lost by the action of those deleterious causes which act injuriously upon all wounds in military hospitals.

When attempts are made to save the limb in what we suppose to be a trivial or doubtful case of knee-joint injury, we should use all of the routine of the antiphlogistic treatment. In a single puncture of the capsule, even when synovia has escaped, the orifice may heal by quick union; but when local inflammation ensues, and runs such an acute course that the free application of leeches—twenty to forty to a limb—do not quell the inflammation, but, running on, we are led to infer that pus has formed within the joint, the articulation should be largely opened, and the joint thoroughly cleansed, whether we resect the heads of the bones or not. There is no longer any injury from the admission of air, whilst there is serious fear of destruction of the cartilages should the collection of pus be retained. This free opening of the articulation may, in some cases, obviate the necessity for secondary resections, as excellent results have been obtained by this apparently bold surgery, the patient saving his life and limb, with an anchylosed joint. The effect of this incision in allaying the general irritation is said to be marked.

The course which will be pursued with a fracture of the bones of the leg must depend upon the extent of injury to the soft parts, and also the facilities at hand for treating fractures. Our main object is always to save life, and, if possible, the limb also; but, in our too-grasping disposition, we must be very guarded how we jeopard the one to save the other. It is in this respect that military surgery is so very different from civil practice, as we are continually compelled to sacrifice limbs to expediency, when, under more favorable conditions, we would not hesitate to practice conservative surgery. To introduce a single example: where a long and tedious transportation becomes necessary after a battle, it would be expedient to amputate much more freely than we would do were hospitals in the immediate neighborhood of the battle field where the wounded could be treated. How, for instance, could we transport with any chance of success a resected joint, such as the shoulder or a gunshot fractured thigh or leg? Under such circumstances an amputation would give the patient a much better chance for life, which should be always the main object.

When facilities offer for attempting the preservation of a fractured leg, the same precautions are taken as in other fractures, for removing immediately all loose or very movable fragments of bone. The limb is placed in a fracture box, or upon the double incline-plane, and by the constant application of cold water, whilst we use those remedies already suggested for keeping down an excessive reaction, we watch the march of the case, and meet the various complications, as they arise, by rules of practice which have been already frequently discussed. Should mortification appear in the wound a few days after the injury, we will find the only means of safety in early amputation.

Resections of the ankle-joint have not been followed by that success which has characterized operations upon the larger joints, especially the knee and the elbow. It is recommended as a conservative practice, but is seldom practiced. When gunshot injuries occur about the ankle, crushing the bones, excision offers but a meagre resource. Mortification often follows upon such injuries, and amputation holds out stronger inducements for immediate and subsequent benefit.

We have often referred to the fact that amputations will ever be a necessity in military surgery; and, according to McLeod, had they been more freely practiced in the Crimea, a larger number of lives would have been saved. It was on that account that, in the distribution of labor, in field infirmaries, it was recommended that the surgeon who had had the greatest experience, and upon whose judgment most reliance could be placed, should officiate as examiner; and his decision should be carried out by those who may possess a greater facility for the operative manual. As a general rule, the following conditions necessitate the loss of a limb, viz: When an entire limb is carried off by a cannon ball, leaving a ragged stump; or when a limb is literally crushed up, although still attached to the body, it will be necessary to amputate to form a good stump; also, if the principal vessels and nerves are torn, even without injury to the bone; or if the soft parts are much lacerated; or in cases of extensive destruction of the skin, as such cases offer very tedious cures if cicatrization is ever obtained; or in severe compound fractures; or often in apparently simple compound fractures, where experience teaches us that although the wound appears trifling to-day, in attempting to save it we will sacrifice a life a few days hence. Amputation is also compulsory when mortification of the limb rapidly follows upon an injury; or when, in compound fractures or perforated joints, the profuse discharge or the continued irritation threatens a fatal issue; also, where joints are crushed, and where resections are not admissible; or where a fracture of the shaft of a bone extends into a joint; or in cases where secondary hemorrhage cannot be controlled by the ligature, or by any other hemostatic. Knowing that in such cases, sooner or later, the limb and life will be jeopardized, we must anticipate these troubles by amputation.

Military surgeons have long made the important division of amputations into primary and secondary—a division of great practical importance, and which forces itself upon our notice by the relative mortality following the two operations. Amputations for direct injury are styled primary; those required for cases of mortification, profuse suppuration, secondary hemorrhage, or for necroses, are called secondary or mediate, and comprise all amputations performed after the first twenty-four or thirty-six hours, when reaction has set in. The experience of every battle field shows, that the mortality following the amputation of limbs which require immediate operation is always less than those performed some days after the infliction of the wound, although the milder cases were those retained, and the most severe those selected for immediate operation. As all military surgeons recognize the propriety of amputating condemned limbs within twenty-four or thirty-six hours after injury, before inflammatory reaction has set in, the subject requires no discussion. The rule in military surgery is absolute, viz: *that the amputating knife should immediately follow the condemnation of the limb.* These are operations for the battle field, and should be performed at the field infirmary. When this golden opportunity, before reaction, is lost, it can never be compensated for.

The rule in performing primary amputations is, to operate as far as possible from the trunk, as every inch diminishes the risk to life. This rule is so general, that when an amputation can be performed at a joint, never amputate higher up; for instance, if an amputation cannot be performed upon the upper part of the leg, remove the limb at the knee-joint rather than amputate the thigh. In secondary amputations it may not be expedient to follow this rule; necessity or the desire to save life, which is always paramount, may compel us to amputate at a distance from the injury, as in cases of mortification. Gangrene should seldom, however, require a secondary amputation, if the rules for primary amputation be followed—of removing at once all limbs in which the blood-vessels and nerves are extensively injured in connection with the crushing of the bones. When mortification attacks a limb, it will be known by the change of color in the skin. When it occurs in the leg, which is its common seat, the foot changes from the natural flesh color to a tallowy or mottled white; the tissues in a measure liquify, are cold, and become offensive—breaking up into more or less extended sloughs, saturated with an ichorous fluid. This gangrenous condition may stop at the ankle, either above or below it, depending upon the seat of injury; or it may creep up to the knee, where it equally shows a disposition to limit its extension. When the ankle limits the mortification, we amputate below the knee; when otherwise, above it. These cases are usually unsatisfactory, as a general poisoning is soon effected, and the stump wherever made, is attacked in a few days, as if by a continuation of the same gangrene.

In mortification of the stump, unless it be in the vicinity of the ankle-joint, a second amputation is not admissible. By the local use of pure nitric acid to the mortified surface, or the concentrated Labarraques' chloride of soda or pyroligneous acid, we strive to limit the extent of the slough; whilst, with carbonate of ammonia, quinine, brandy, and strong food, we support the system until some improvement makes its appearance in the stump. When all the sloughs have been eliminated and the stump has commenced to cicatrize, will be time enough to remodel the old amputation, by cutting off the protruding bone, which is always better than performing a second amputation.

Having condemned a limb, we should wait until the nervous shock—from which most of the wounded suffer—subsides, and then give chloroform. Should we not have the time for its proper inhalation, we may inject a half grain or more of morphine under the skin, which will produce a rapid blunting of nervous sensibilities; and in five minutes, or even in less time, the patient will be in a fit condition to stand the operation, with the least degree of constitutional shock.

In the performance of all serious operations, when possible, there should be three assistants. One aid gives the chloroform; a second compresses the main artery, which is much better than using the tourniquet—an instrument which is now in a great measure discarded from practice; and a third holds the limb and supports the flap during the section. The aid who administered the chloroform during the incisions, can assist in ligating the arteries. Military surgeons prefer the circular operation to the flap, which they only use in the exceptional cases. With the circular stump, covered only by skin, there is less soft tissue to suppurate and slough, and a much more rapid cicatrization is effected. Experience, which has long recognized the utility of the circular operation for the leg, has now generalized it as the most useful amputation for the thigh or arm.

Having assigned the aids their posts, and seen that all the necessary instruments which may be needed are at hand—for a surgeon should never commence an operation until he has satisfied himself on this score—the surgeon removes the limb, ligates the vessels, and when all oozing has ceased, secures the stump by points of suture placed at intervals of an inch or a little less along the entire line of wound.

In dividing the skin, the surgeon cannot be too careful to leave an ample flap to cover the heads of the bones. This is the first and most important rule in amputation. You cannot well leave too much skin, and can very easily commit the opposite error. The surplus of skin will be absorbed; a deficiency can in no way be supplied. The rule is, to have the flaps so ample that no tension be necessary in closing the wound. One of the most constant as well as one of the most frightful exhibitions in military hospitals, where the surgeons have not yet gained experience, is the protrusion of the bones from the stumps of amputated limbs, necessitating a second operation, should the patient survive the first. A little care will obviate all of this trouble, and save the surgeon much mortification. Any omission in this respect must be corrected before the stump is dressed; and if the bone is found so long that the skin cannot be made to cover it without traction, remove a section of bone with the saw, and not attempt, through want of honesty, to conceal a badly-performed operation, and make the innocent patient the victim of our misplaced pride. In ligating the vessels, tie every one which bleeds or is likely to bleed. It is not derogatory for a surgeon to apply ten, fifteen, or even twenty ligatures to a stump; it shows that he understands his profession; experience has taught him the great trouble and annoyance of reopening a stump to find a bleeding vessel, when he has but little time to attend to the urgent demands of the wounded. *The rule is, neglect no small artery.*

As adhesive straps for supporting and sustaining the flaps are antagonistic to water dressings, they are useless in amputations, and are not used, except a small patch to secure the ligatures upon the limb at one angle of the wound. A single layer of wet cloth is applied to the stump; this in turn is covered by a piece of waxed cloth, to keep in the moisture, and either an ice bladder or water by irrigation is continuously applied over this outer cloth. The case should now be looked upon as a wound, and should be treated accordingly. The course laid down for wounds is here strictly applicable, and should be closely followed. Sutures are recommended in all operations, as they keep the flaps in apposition, not being influenced by the water dressings; they also obviate much after-dressing. The use of sutures does away with adhesive straps, which, when water dressings are used, are always inconvenient and often useless.

In certain cases of amputation, as in the circular, where the skin alone forms the flap, the dressing may be changed, as follows: After applying sutures to the entire length of the wound, draw the intervening spaces accurately together by means of strips of isinglass plaster, and cover, also, the length of the wound with a folded strip, only leaving uncovered the angle where the ligatures escape and where drainage from within is permitted. The object of the dressing is to convert the wound into a subcutaneous one, excluding the air and hastening union. To the stump no other dressing is applied, the wound being exposed. No water dressing is to be used, and the stump is left unmolested, except cleansing the effects of drainage; when, at the expiration of a week, the removal of the straps will complete cicatrization along the line of incision. In healthy patients and in a pure atmosphere, a rapid healing of stumps may in this way be obtained. The isinglass plaster will alone answer—

the diachylon being too irritating and not sufficiently pliant to seal hermetically the wound. We find but little use for ointments in dressing stumps, the wet cloth being much simpler, not irritating, and therefore more efficient.

During the treatment of all wounds in military hospitals, previous want and exposure, which belongs to every army, however well organized, will show their influence; and if the plan of abstemious or antiphlogistic diet be adopted for those operated upon, from misguided views of the pathology of inflammation, the mortality will be heavy. Liberal feeding tells in the after-treatment of amputations; and the great difference in the surgical statistics of the French and English depends more perhaps upon the diet in their hospital practice than upon any one other cause. Tisanes cannot support a person in ordinary health, and certainly cannot support him under the additional drain of an exhausting suppuration. If patients are placed under identically similar conditions, the successful treatment of amputations will be found to lean to the side of those who are the most liberally supported. Slops are out of place in a surgical hospital, and good cooking will be found as useful as good nursing. Let nature be our guide. For the first one or two days after a serious operation there is but little disposition to eat. Under such conditions, I would not advise food to be forced; but as soon as the patient expresses a desire to eat, foster his appetite with good, strong, nourishing, easily-digested food, and let his supply be liberal. Any attempt at starvation will be highly injurious.

If the patient escapes the ordinary diseases incident to hospitals, viz: erysipelas, gangrene, pyæmia, etc., we must be extremely careful of him about the tenth or twelfth day. When the ligatures are escaping from the arteries, absolute rest should be insisted upon, and the patient should not be allowed to exert himself in any way until this fear of secondary hemorrhage is passed. We have elsewhere stated how this complication is to be met.

Whenever operations are to be performed in military surgery, *chloroform* should be administered. It is a remedy which the surgeon should never be without, and which might be used on all occasions with advantage; whether for operations or for dressing painful wounds, as in the cleansing of compound fractures. The effects of chloroform are wonderful in mitigating the suffering of the wounded, and it is often instrumental in the cure of wounds, from the rest and tranquility of mind which follows its inhalation. It also prevents excessive reaction in the paroxysms of traumatic fever. During the performance of capital operations on the battle field, death sometimes ensues from nervous exhaustion, produced by excess of suffering; the use of chloroform relieves the patient at least from this risk. Those brought up in the older school, before the days of anæsthetics, in refusing all innovations, still insist on decrying the dangers of this potent remedy, and moralize upon the duty of suffering, as submitting to an express infliction from on high. Although the French surgeons in the Crimea report the successful administration of chloroform to thirty thousand wounded, without a single accident, and McLeod refers to its great utility in the Crimea, where it was administered to twenty thousand soldiers, and more than realized the most enthusiastic anticipations of the medical staffs, still we find some of the older school, who are in authority, sneer at its pretensions and magnify its dangers. Dr. Hall, who is at the head of the English medical staff, in giving instructions to the surgeons upon entering active service in the Crimea, cautioned them against the administration of chloroform in the severe shock of serious gunshot wounds, as he thinks that few will survive where it is used. But as he finds public opinion, which he calls mistaken philanthropy, against him, he disparages chloroform, and lauds the lusty bawling of the wounded from the smart of the knife, as a powerful stimulant which has roused many a sinking man from his apathetic state. Some of the older surgeons characterize the cries of the patient as music to the ear, and speak of it as an advantage to be courted, and not to be suppressed. Notwithstanding such advice, the universal use of chloroform in the Crimea and later in Italy, is a complete vindication of the utility of the remedy, and proof of its necessity: and now we consider it an essential among army supplies. For ourselves, who place unlimited confidence in its judicious administration, and, with a large experience, we have never had the slightest cause to doubt its advantages under every circumstance. We hope that the humanizing tendencies of the age, in introducing this invaluable comfort, has banished that dread of being cut as an item to be considered when operations are necessary; and we hope to see anæsthetics used as liberally in allaying the pain of surgical affections as cold water is now used for keeping down inflammation. *We do not hesi-*

tate to say, that it should be given to every patient requiring a serious or painful operation. We may hear now and then of an accident from its administration, but who can tell us of the immense number who would have sunk from operations, had it not been administered?

In its administration we must use the following precautions: The best apparatus is a folded cloth in a form of a cone, in the apex of which a small piece of sponge is placed. This is first held at some distance from the nose and mouth of the patient, so that the first inhalation may be well diluted with air. As the exhilarating stage is reached, the cloth should be approached to the nose, so that a more concentrated ether may be inhaled, which will rapidly produce the desired insensibility. Noisy breathing is the sign that the anæsthetic effect is produced, when the inhalation should be suspended and the operation commenced. Unless the operation is very tedious, do not renew the inhalation.

Ingenious inhalors are more or less complicated, and are on that account more or less inefficient. The great perfection of the above-mentioned apparatus is its simplicity. Finding that much chloroform is wasted by evaporation from the handkerchief, I have for some years used a common funnel as my inhalor, which protects the hands of the person administering the chloroform, and prevents the loss from general evaporation. If a piece of heavy wire or a small bar of tin be attached across the interior of the funnel, about half-way toward its throat, the sponge containing the chloroform can be supported between this bar and the side of the funnel, leaving a space on one side for the air to rush over the surface of the sponge as it comes through the elongated end of the apparatus, when the air loaded with ether is inhaled. The funnel should be large enough to cover the lower half of the face, including nose and mouth, and the sponge should not come within two inches of the face, for should it touch the skin it would blister it. The eyes, being excluded from the apparatus, are not annoyed by the evaporation of chloroform. As the funnel does not fit accurately to the lower outline of the face, there will be ample spaces on either side of the chin to admit air for diluting the vapor. Besides a great saving of chloroform, which is no small recommendation, the use of this instrument obviates the fear of suffocation, which is always present to my mind when I see chloroform carelessly administered. When the cloth is used, should the patient struggle—a very common occurrence—or should the assistant administering the anæsthetic be at all interested in the operation, the cloth is thrust down upon the face of the patient, respiration is impeded, and suffocation is imminent. Suppose the patient has already been influenced to such an extent that he has lost the voluntary control of his muscles, and cannot pull away the cloth, he is in a very dangerous condition, and the continued thoughtlessness of the assistant might suffocate him. I can readily understand, in this way, why deaths should sometimes occur from the carelessness of administration, and am only surprised that it occurs so seldom. Were we as careless in the use of other potent remedies as we are of chloroform, cases of poisoning would be largely increased. In times of hurry, confusion and excitement, as after a battle, we cannot surround the safety and well-being of the wounded with too many guards for their protection.

APPENDIX.

Appendix No. 1.

REGULATIONS
FOR
THE MEDICAL DEPARTMENT
OF THE
CONFEDERATE STATES.

1.... The *Surgeon-General* is charged with the administrative details of the medical department, the government of hospitals, the regulation of the duties of surgeons and assistant surgeons, and the appointment of acting medical officers, when needed, for local or detached service. He will issue orders and instructions relating to the professional duties of medical officers; and all communications from them, which require his action, will be made directly to him.

2.... The senior medical officer on duty with an army corps in the field, is the *Medical Director* of that army, and he will have the general control of the medical officers.

3.... The medical director will inspect the hospitals under his control, and see that the rules and regulations with regard to them and the duties of the surgeons and assistant surgeons, are enforced.

4.... He will examine the case books, prescription and diet books, and ascertain the nature of diseases which may have prevailed, and their probable causes; recommend the best method of prevention, and also make such suggestions relative to the situation, construction and economy of the hospitals, as may appear necessary for the benefit and comfort of the sick and the good of the service.

5....He will require from the medical officers of the command monthly reports of the sick and wounded (Form 1), and from the data furnished by them, will make to the Surgeon-General a consolidated monthly report of the sick and wounded.

6....He will make to the Surgeon-General a monthly return (Form 2) of the medical officers of the command.

7....The *Medical Purveyors* will, under the direction of the Surgeon-General, purchase all medical and hospital supplies required for the medical department of the army.

8....Medical purveyors will make to the Surgeon-General, at the end of each fiscal quarter, returns in duplicate (Form 3) of medical supplies received, issued and remaining on hand, stating to whom, or from whom, and when and where issued or received. Other medical officers in charge of medical supplies will make similar returns semi-annually, on the 30th of June and the 31st of December: and all medical officers will make them when relieved from the duty to which their returns relate. The returns will show the condition of the stores, and particularly of the instruments, bedding and furniture. Medical purveyors will furnish abstracts of receipts and issues with their returns (Form 4).

9....Medical disbursing officers will, at the end of each fiscal quarter, render to the Surgeon-General, in duplicate, a quarterly account current of moneys received and expended, with the proper vouchers for the payments, and certificates that the services have been rendered and the supplies purchased and received for the medical service, and transmit to him an estimate of the funds required for the next quarter.

10....The medical supplies for the army are prescribed in the Standard Supply Tables for Hospitals or Field Service.

11....Medical and hospital supplies will be obtained by making requisitions, in duplicate (Form 5), on the Surgeon-General, forwarding them through the medical director of the command. If an army be in the field, and there be a medical purveyor in charge of supplies, requisitions will be made on him, after receiving the approval of the medical director.

12....When it is necessary to purchase medical supplies, and recourse cannot be had to a medical disbursing officer, they may be procured by the quartermaster on a special requisition (Form 6) and account (Form 7).

13....In every case of *special* requisition, a duplicate of the requisition shall, at the same time, be transmitted to the Surgeon-General, for his information.

14....An officer transferring medical supplies, will furnish a certified invoice to the officer who is to receive them, and transmit a duplicate of it to the Surgeon-General. The receiving officer will transmit duplicate receipts to the Surgeon-General, with a report of the quality and condition of the supplies, and report the same to the issuing officer. A medical officer who turns over medical supplies to a quartermaster for storage or transportation, will forward to the Surgeon-General, with the invoice, the quartermaster's receipts for the packages.

15....Medical officers will take up and account for all medical supplies of the army that come into their possession, and report, when they know it, to whose account they are to be credited.

16....In all official lists of medical supplies, the articles will be entered in the order of the supply table.

17....The senior medical officer of a hospital will distribute the patients, according to convenience and the nature of their complaints, into wards or divisions, under the particular charge of the several assistant surgeons, and will visit them himself each day as frequently as the state of the sick may require, accompanied by the assistant, steward and nurse.

18....His prescriptions of medicine and diet are written down at once in the proper register, with the name of the patient and the number of his bed; the assistants fill up the diet table for the day, and direct the administration of the prescribed medicines. He will detail an assistant surgeon to remain at the hospital day and night, when the state of the sick requires it.

19....In distributing the duties of his assistants, he will ordinarily require the aid of one in the care and preparation of the hospital reports, registers and records, the rolls and descriptive lists; and of another, in the charge of the dispensary, instruments, medicines, hospital expenditures, and the preparation of the requisitions and annual returns.

20....He will enforce the proper hospital regulations to promote health and prevent contagion, by ventilated and not crowded rooms, scrupulous cleanliness, frequent changes of bedding and linen, occasional refilling of the bed sacks and pillow ticks with fresh straw, regularity in meals, attention to cooking, etc.

21....He will require the steward to take due care of the hospital stores and supplies; to enter in a book, daily (Form 8), the issues to the wardmasters, cooks and nurses; to prepare the provision returns, and receive and distribute the rations.

22....He will require the wardmaster to take charge of the effects of the patients; to register them in a book (Form 9); to have them numbered and labelled with the patient's name, rank and company; to receive from the steward the furniture, bedding, cooking utensils, etc., for use, and keep a record of them (Form 10), and how distributed to the wards and kitchens, and once a week to take an inventory of the articles in use, and report to him any loss or damage to them, and to return to the steward such as are not required for use.

23....Assistant surgeons will obey the orders of their senior surgeon; see that subordinate officers do their duty, and aid in enforcing the regulations of the hospital.

24....The cooks and nurses are under the orders of the steward. He is responsible for the cleanliness of the wards and kitchens, patients and attendants, and all articles in use. He will ascertain who are present at sunrise and sunset, and tattoo, and report absentees.

25....At surgeon's call the sick then in the companies will be conducted to the hospital by the first sergeants, who will each hand to the surgeon, in his company book, a list of all the sick of the company, on which the surgeon shall state who are to remain or go into hospital; who are to return to quarters as sick or convalescent; what duties the convalescents in quarters are capable of; what cases are feigned; and any other information in regard to the sick of the company he may have to communicate to the company commander.

26....Soldiers in hospital, patients or attendants, except stewards, shall be mustered on the rolls of their company, if it be present at the post.

27....When a soldier in hospital is detached from his company so as not to be mustered with it for pay, his company commander shall certify and send to the hospital his descriptive list, and account of pay and clothing, containing all necessary information relating to his accounts with the Government, on which the surgeon shall enter all payments, stoppages, and issues of clothing to him in hospital. When he leaves the hospital, the medical officer shall certify and remit his descriptive list, showing the state of his accounts. If he is discharged from the service in hospital, the surgeon shall make out his final statements for pay and clothing. If he dies in hospital, the surgeon shall take charge of his effects, and make the reports required in the general regulations concerning soldiers who die absent from their companies.

28....Patients in hospitals are, if possible, to leave their arms and accoutrements with their companies, and in no case to take ammunition into the hospital.

29....When a patient is transferred from one hospital to another, the medical officer shall send with him an account of his case and the treatment.

30....The regulations for the service of hospitals apply, as far as practicable, to the medical service in the field.

31....The senior medical officer of each hospital, post, regiment or detachment, will keep the following records, and deliver them to his successor: A register of patients (Form 11); a prescription and diet book (Form 12); a case book; copies of his requisitions, annual returns, and reports of sick and wounded; and an order and letter book; in which will be transcribed all orders and letters relating to his duties.

32....He will make the muster and pay rolls of the hospital steward and matrons, and of all soldiers in hospital, sick or on duty, detached from their companies, on the forms furnished from the Adjutant-General's office, and according to the directions expressed on them.

33....The extra pay allowed to soldiers acting as cooks and nurses in hospitals, will be paid by the pay department. Such extra services will be noted on the hospital muster rolls, and for the sums thus expended the pay department will be reimbursed by the medical department.

34....The senior medical officer will select the cooks, nurses and matrons, with the approval of the commanding officer. Cooks and nurses will be taken from the privates, and will be exempt from other duty, but shall attend the parades for muster and weekly inspection of their companies at the post, unless specially excused by the commanding officer.

35....Ordinarily, hospital attendants are allowed as follows: To a general hospital, one steward, one nurse as wardmaster, one nurse to ten patients, one matron to twenty, and one cook to thirty; to a hospital, where the command exceeds five companies, one steward and wardmaster, one cook, two matrons, and four nurses; to a post or garrison of one company, one steward and wardmaster, one nurse, one cook, and one matron; and for every two companies more, one nurse; at arsenals, where the number of enlisted men is not less than fourteen, one matron is allowed. The allowance of hospital attendants for a regiment in the field will be, for one company, one steward, one nurse and one cook; for each additional company, one nurse; and for command of over five companies, one additional cook.

36....Medical officers, where on duty, will attend the officers and enlisted men, and the servants and laundresses authorized by law; and at stations where other medical attendance cannot be procured, and on marches, the hired men of the army. Medicines will be dispensed to the families of officers and soldiers, and to all persons entitled to medical attendance; hospital stores to enlisted men.

37....Medical officers, in giving certificates of disability (Form 13), are to take particular care in all cases that have not been under their charge; and especially in epilepsy, convulsions, chronic rheumatism, derangement of the urinary organs, ophthalmia, ulcers, or any obscure disease, liable to be feigned or purposely produced; and in no case shall such certificate be given until after sufficient time and examination to detect any attempt at deception.

38....In passing a recruit, the medical officer is to examine him stripped; to see that he has free use of all of his limbs; that his chest is ample; that his hearing, vision and speech are perfect; that he has no tumors, or ulcerated or extensively cicatrized legs; no rupture, or chronic cutaneous affection; that he has not received any contusion or wound of the head that may impair his faculties; that he is not a drunkard; is not subject to convulsions, and has no infectious disorder, nor any other that may unfit him for military service.

39....As soon as a recruit joins any regiment or station, he shall be examined by the medical officer, and vaccinated when it is required.

40....Medical officers attending recruiting rendezvous, will keep a record (Form 18) of all the recruits examined by them. Books for this purpose will be procured by application to the Surgeon-General, to whom they will be returned when filled.

41....The senior medical officer of each hospital, post, regiment or detachment, will make monthly to the medical director, and quarterly to the Surgeon-General, a report of sick and wounded, and of deaths, and of certificates for discharge for disability (Form 1).

42....After surgeon's call, he will make a morning report of the sick to the commanding officer (Form 14).

43....Every medical officer will report to the Surgeon-General and to the medical director the date when he arrives at a station, or when he leaves it, and his orders in the case, and at the end of each month, whenever not at his station, whether on service or on leave of absence; and when on leave of absence, his post-office address for the next month. They will also acknowledge the receipt of all orders.

44....When medical attendance is required by officers or enlisted men on service, or for the authorized servants of such officers, and the attendance of a medical officer cannot be had, the officer, or if there be no officer, then the enlisted man, may employ a private physician, and a just account therefor will be paid by the medical bureau.

45....The account will set out the name of the patient, the date of and charge for each visit, and for medicines. The physician will make a certificate to the account in case of an officer, or affidavit in case of an enlisted man, that the account is correct, and the charges are the customary charges of the place.

46....The officer will make his certificate, or the enlisted man his affidavit, to the correctness of the account, that he was on service at the place, and stating the circumstances preventing him from receiving the services of a medical officer.

47....When the charge is against an officer, he will pay the account if practicable, and transmit it to the medical bureau for reimbursement. In all other cases, the account will be transmitted to the medical bureau for settlement.

48....If the charge is against a deceased officer or enlisted man, the physician will make the affidavit, before required, to the account, and that he has been paid no part of it.

49....No charges for consultation fees will be paid by the medical bureau; nor will any account for medical attendance or medicines be paid, if the officer or enlisted man be not on service.

50....When it is necessary to employ a private physician as medical officer, the commanding officer may do it by written contract, conditioned as in Form 15, at a stated compensation, not to exceed $50 a month, when the number of officers and men, with authorized servants and laundresses, is one hundred or more; $40 when it is from fifty to one hundred, and $30 when it is under fifty.

51....But when he is required to abandon his own business, and give his whole time to the public service, the contract may be not to exceed $80 a month; and not to exceed $100, besides transportation in kind to be furnished by the Quartermaster's Department, where he is required to accompany troops on marches or transports. But a private physician will not be employed to accompany troops on marches or transports, except by orders from the War Department, or in particular and urgent cases, by the order of the officer directing the movement; when a particular statement of the circumstances which made it necessary will be appended to the contract.

52....And when a private physician is required to furnish medicines, he will be allowed, besides the liquidated pay, from twenty-five to fifty per cent. on it, to be determined by the Surgeon-General.

53....In all cases a duplicate of the contract will be transmitted forthwith by the commanding officer to the Surgeon-General; and the commanding officer for the time being will at once discontinue it whenever the necessity for it ceases, or the Surgeon-General may so direct.

54....The physician's account of pay due must be sent to the Surgeon-General for payment, vouched by the certificate of the commanding officer, that it is correct and agreeable to contract, and that the services have been duly rendered. But when it cannot be conveniently submitted to the Surgeon-General from the frontier or the field, it may be paid on the order of the commanding officer, not to exceed the regular amount, by a medical disbursing officer or a quartermaster.

55.... The General-in-Chief will appoint, on the recommendation of the Surgeon-General, from the enlisted men of the army, or cause to be enlisted, as many competent hospital stewards as the service may require.

56....As the hospital stewards are "attached to the Medical Department," their accounts of pay, clothing, etc., must be kept by the medical officers under whose immediate direction they are serving, who are also responsible for certified statements of such accounts, and correct descriptive lists of such stewards, to accompany them in case of transfer; as, also, that their final statements and certificates of discharge are accurately made out, when they are at length discharged from service.

57....The senior medical officer of a command requiring a steward may recommend a competent non-commissioned officer or soldier to be appointed, which recommendation the commanding officer shall forward to the Adjutant-General of the army, with his remarks thereon, and with the remarks of the company commander.

58....When no competent enlisted man can be procured,

the medical officer will report the fact to the Surgeon-General. Applications and testimonials of competency, from persons seeking to be enlisted for hospital stewards, may be addressed to the Surgeon-General.

59....No soldier or citizen will be recommended for appointment, who is not *known* to be temperate, honest, and in every way reliable, as well as sufficiently intelligent, and skilled in pharmacy, for the proper discharge of the responsible duties likely to be devolved upon him. Until this is *known*, he will be appointed as acting steward by the medical officer, with the approval of the commanding officer.

60....Hospital stewards, appointed by the General-in-Chief, whenever stationed in places whence no post return is made to the Adjutant-General's office, or when on furlough, will, at the end of every month, report themselves, by letter, to the Adjutant-General and Surgeon-General, as well as to the medical director of the military department in which they may be serving; to each of whom they will also report each new assignment to duty, or change of station, ordered in their case, noting carefully the number, date and source of the order directing the same. They will likewise report monthly, when on furlough, to the medical officer in charge of the hospital to which they are attached.

61....The jurisdiction and authority of courts-martial are the same with reference to hospital stewards as in the cases of other enlisted men. When, however, a hospital steward is sentenced by an inferior court to be reduced to the ranks, such sentence, though it may be approved by the reviewing officer, will not be carried into effect until the case has been referred to the General-in-Chief for final action. In these cases of reduction, the application of the man for discharge from service, though not recognized as of right, will generally be regarded with favor, if his offence has not been of too serious a nature, and especially when he has not been recently promoted from the ranks.

[It is urged that medical officers make requisition only for such medicines in the following table as are deemed indispensable.]

Standard Supply Table for General and Post Hospitals.

ARTICLES.	Quantities for one year for commands of				
	From 100 to 200.	From 200 to 300.	From 300 to 400.	500 men.	1,000 men.
MEDICINES.					
Acaciæ ....lb..	2	4	6	8	16
Acidi acetici ....lb..	½	1	2	*2½	5
" arseniosi.............oz..	½	1	2	2½	5
" benzoici ....oz..	1	2	3	4	8
" citrici ....lb..	1	2	3	4	8
" muriatici ....lb..	½	1	2	2½	5
" nitrici ....lb..	1	2	3	4	8
" sulphurici............lb..	1	2	3	4	8
" " aromatici....lb..	1	2	3	4	8
" tannici ....oz..	2	4	6	8	16
" tartarici ....lb..	2	4	6	8	16
Ætheris sulphurici loti......lb..	2	4	6	8	16
Alcoholis ....bott..	24	48	72	96	192
Aluminis ....lb..	1	2	3	4	8
Ammoniacia ....lb..	½	1	2	2½	5
Ammoniæ carbonatis ....oz..	8	16	24	32	64
" muriatis ....lb..	½	1	2	2½	5
Anthemidis ....lb..	1	2	3	4	8
Antimonii et potass. tartratis.oz..	3	6	9	12	24
Argenti nitratis (crystals)....oz..	1	2	3	4	8
" " (fused) .....oz..	1	2	3	4	8
Arnicæ.....................lb..	1	2	3	4	8
Assafœtidæ ....oz..	4	8	12	16	32
Bismuthi subnitratis.........oz..	4	8	12	16	32
Camphoræ..................lb..	2	4	6	8	16
Cardamomi ....oz..	8	16	24	32	64
Catechu ....lb..	½	1	2	2½	5
Ceræ albæ*....... ....lb..	2	4	6	8	16
Cerati resinæ ... .lb..	2	4	6	8	16
" zimplicis ....lb..	8	16	24	32	64
" zinci carbonatis ......lb..	2	4	6	8	16
Chloroformi................lb..	1	2	3	4	8
Collodii ....oz..	2	4	6	8	16
Copaibæ....................lb..	5	10	15	20	40
Creasoti ....oz..	2	4	6	8	16
Cretæ preparatæ ....lb..	1	2	3	4	8
Cupri sulphatis ....oz..	2	4	6	8	16
Emplastri adhæsivi ....yds..	5	10	15	20	40
" cantharadis ......lb..	3	6	9	12	24

*To be issued to posts where simple cerate cannot be sent without becoming rancid.

SUPPLY TABLE FOR HOSPITALS—Continued.

ARTICLES.	Quantities for one year for commands of				
	From 100 to 200.	From 200 to 300.	From 300 to 400.	500 men.	1,000 men.
Emplastri ferri ....lb..	1	2	3	4	8
" hydrargyri.......lb..	½	1	2	2½	5
" ichthyocollæ.. .yds..	3	6	9	12	24
Extracti belladonnæ........oz..	2	4	6	8	16
" buchu fluidi.......lb..	1	2	3	4	8
" colchici acetici ....oz..	1	2	3	4	8
" colocynthidis comp..oz..	8	16	24	32	64
" colombæ fluidi.....lb..	1	2	3	4	8
" conii ....oz..	1	2	3	4	8
" cubebæ fluidi......lb..	1	2	3	4	8
" gentianæ fluidi ....lb..	1	2	3	4	8
" glycyrrhizæ ....lb..	6	12	18	24	48
" hyoscyami ....oz..	2	4	6	8	16
" ipecacuanhæ fluidi.lb..	½	1	2	2½	5
" piperis fluidi ......oz..	1	2	3	4	8
" pruni virg. fluidi...lb..	1	2	3	4	8
" rhei fluidi ....lb..	1	2	3	4	8
" sarsaparillæ fluidi..lb..	2	4	6	8	16
" senegæ fluidi ......lb..	½	1	2	2½	5
" sennæ fluidi.......lb..	1	2	3	4	8
" taraxaci fluidi.....lb..	1	2	3	4	8
" valerianæ fluidi .. .oz..	8	16	24	32	64
" zingiberis fluidi....lb..	½	1	2	2½	5
Ferri iodidi...............oz..	2	4	6	8	16
" et quiniæ citratis......oz..	4	8	12	16	32
" sulphatis............oz..	2	4	6	8	16
Gambogiæ................oz..	½	1	2	2½	5
Glycerine.................oz..	2	4	6	8	16
Guaiaci resinæ............lb..	½	1	2	2½	5
Hydrargyri chloridi corr....oz..	½	1	2	2½	5
" " mitis...lb..	1	2	3	4	8
" cum cretâ ... ..lb..	½	1	2	2½	5
" iodidi..........oz..	1	2	3	4	8
" oxidi rubri .....oz..	1	2	3	4	8
Iodinii....................oz..	2	4	6	8	16
Lini......................lb..	4	8	12	16	32
Liquoris ammoniæ ....lb..	4	8	12	16	32
" ferri iodidi ....lb..	1	2	3	4	8
" potass: arsenitis ...oz..	2	4	6	8	16
" sodæ chlorinatæ...bott..	3	6	9	12	24
" zinci chloridi ....bott..	3	6	9	12	24
Magnesiæ ....lb..	½	1	2	2½	5
" sulphatis........ lb..	25	50	75	100	200
Massæ pill: hydrargyri .....oz..	8	16	24	32	64
Mellis despumati ....lb..	2	4	6	8	16
Morphiæ sulphatis ....dr..	2	4	6	8	16

SUPPLY TABLE FOR HOSPITALS—Continued.

ARTICLES.	Quantities for one year for commands of				
	From 100 to 200.	From 200 to 300.	From 300 to 400.	500 men.	1,000 men.
Myrrhæ ....lb..	½	1	2	2½	5
Olei anisi....................oz..	1	2	3	4	8
" cajuputi ....oz..	1	2	3	4	8
" caryophylli ....oz..	1	2	3	4	8
" cinnamomi............oz..	1	2	3	4	8
" menthæ piperitæ ......oz..	2	4	6	8	16
" morrhuæ ....bott..	8	16	24	32	64
" olivæ ....bott..	8	16	24	32	64
" origani ....oz..	4	8	12	16	32
" ricini............qt. bott..	12	24	36	48	96
" terebinthinæ .....qt. bott..	4	8	12	16	32
" tiglii ....dr..	2	4	6	8	16
Opii.........................lb..	½	1	2	2½	5
Picis abietis ....lb..	1	2	3	4	8
Plumbi acetatis ....lb..	1	2	3	4	8
Potassæ acetatis............lb..	1	2	3	4	8
" bicarbonatis........lb..	1	2	3	4	8
" bitartratis..........lb..	2	4	6	8	16
" chloratis ....lb..	1	2	3	4	8
" nitratis.............lb..	1	2	3	4	8
" sulphatis...........lb..	½	1	2	2½	5
Potassii cyanureti..........dr..	1	2	3	4	8
" iodidi................oz..	8	16	24	32	64
Pruni virginianæ...........lb..	½	1	2	2½	5
Pulveris acaciæ ....lb..	2	4	6	8	16
" aloës...............oz..	4	8	12	16	32
" cantharidis........oz..	2	4	6	8	16
" capsici............lb..	1	2	3	4	8
" cinchonæ ....lb..	1	2	3	4	8
" ferri...............oz..	2	4	6	8	16
" " per sulphatis ..oz..	1	2	3	4	8
" glycyrrhizæ ....oz..	4	8	12	16	32
" ipecacuanhæ.......lb..	½	1	2	2½	5
" " et opii.lb..	½	1	2	2½	5
" jalapæ ....oz..	4	8	12	16	32
" lini ....lb..	8	16	24	32	64
" opii.... ....lb..	½	1	2	2½	5
" rhei...............oz..	4	8	12	16	32
" sabinæ............oz..	1	2	3	4	8
" sinapis nigræ......lb..	6	12	18	24	48
" ulmi ....lb..	2	4	6	8	16
Quassiæ ....lb..	½	1	2	2½	5
Quiniæ sulphatis...........oz..	10–20	20–40	30–60	40–80	80–160
Rhei ....oz..	4	8	12	16	32
Sacchari...................lb..	20	40	60	80	160
Saponis ....lb..	4	8	12	16	32

SUPPLY TABLE FOR HOSPITALS—Continued.

ARTICLES.	Quantities for one year for commands of				
	From 100 to 200.	From 200 to 300.	From 300 to 400.	500 men.	1,000 men.
Scillæ.......................oz..	4	8	12	16	32
Serpentariæ...............lb..	½	1	2	2½	5
Sodæ bicarbonatis..........lb..	2	4	6	8	16
" boratis...............lb..	½	1	2	2½	5
" et potass: tartratis ...lb..	3	6	9	12	24
Spigeliæ...................lb..	½	1	2	2½	5
Spiritus ammon: aromatici..oz..	2	4	6	8	16
" ætheris compositi...lb..	½	1	2	2½	5
" " nitrici......lb..	2	4	6	8	16
" lavandulæ comp....lb..	½	1	2	2½	5
" vini gallici.......bott..	12	24	36	48	96
Strychniæ ....dr..	1	2	3	4	8
Sulphuris loti..............lb..	1	2	3	4	8
Syrupi scillæ..............lb..	3	6	9	12	24
Tincturæ aconiti radicis ....lb..	1	2	3	4	8
" digitalis..........oz..	4	8	12	16	32
" ergotæ (Dublin).. oz..	4	8	12	16	32
" ferri chloridi......lb..	½	1	2	2½	5
" veratri viridis ....oz..	4	8	12	16	32
Unguenti hydrargyri ....lb..	1	2	3	4	8
" " nitratis.lb..	½	1	2	2½	5
Veratriæ.................dr..	1	2	3	4	8
Vini colchici seminis........lb..	½	1	2	2½	5
Zinci acetatis..............oz..	1	2	3	4	8
" sulphatis.............oz..	1	2	3	4	8
" chlorid............. oz..	½	1	1	2	3
INSTRUMENTS.					
Buck's spongeholder for the throat ....no..	1	1	1	1	1
Cupping glasses or tins.....no..	12	12	18	18	24
Dissecting..............sets..	1	1	1	1	1
Lancets, spring*...........no..	1	1	2	2	4
" thumb†........ ..no..	4	6	8	8	12
Obstetrical ....sets..	1	1	1	1	1
Pocket...................sets..	1	1	1	1	1
Probangs ....no..	6	6	6	6	6
Pulleys ....sets..	1	1	1	1	1
Scarificators..............no..	2	2	2	3	4
Splints (assorted).........sets..	1	1	1	1	2
Stethoscopes.... ....no..	1	1	1	1	1
Stomach pump and case ....no..	1	1	1	1	1
Syringes, enema‡..........no..	3	3	3	3	6

* Four extra fleams to each lancet. † With cases. ‡ 1 Davidson's: 1, 4-oz.: 1, 8-oz.

ARTICLES.	Quantities for one year for commands of				
	From 100 to 200.	From 200 to 300.	From 300 to 400.	500 men.	1,000 men.
Syringes, penis, glass.......no..	2	4	6	8	16
" " metallic....no..	6	12	18	24	36
" vagina*..........no..	3	3	3	3	6
Teeth extracting.........sets..	1	1	1	1	2
Tongue depressor (hinge)...no..	1	1	1	1	2
Tourniquets, field..........no..	4	4	6	6	10
" spiral.........no..	1	1	2	2	4
Trusses, herniæ............no..	3	6	9	12	24
BOOKS.					
Anatomy ....cop..	1	1	1	1	1
Chemistry................cop..	1	1	1	1	1
Dispensatory ....cop..	1	1	1	1	1
Medical Dictionary ....cop..	1	1	1	1	1
" Formulary........cop..	1	1	1	1	1
" Jurisprudence and Toxicology .....cop..	1	1	1	1	1
" Practice..........cop..	1	1	1	1	1
Obstetricy................cop..	1	1	1	1	1
Regulations for Med. Dep't.cop..	1	1	1	2	2
Surgery..................cop..	1	1	1	1	1
Blank ....no..	2	2	2	3	4
Case.....................no..	1	1	1	1	1
Meteorological Register ....no..	1	1	1	1	1
Order and Letter ....no..	1	1	1	1	1
Prescription..............no..	1	1	1	1	1
Register ....no..	1	1	1	1	1
Requisitions, Returns, Reports of sick } ....no..	1	1	1	1	1
HOSPITAL STORES.					
Arrowroot ....lb..	5	10	15	20	40
Barley ....lb..	20	40	60	80	160
Cinnamon ....lb..	½	1	2	2½	5
Cloves ....oz..	4	8	12	16	32
Cocoa ....lb..	10	20	30	40	80
Farina ....lb..	5	10	15	20	40
Ginger, ground (Jamaica)...lb..	½	1	2	2½	5
Nutmegs ....oz..	4	8	12	16	32
Tea......................lb..	20	40	60	80	160
Whiskey, bottles of........doz..	2	4	6	8	16

* Hard india-rubber, 1; glass, 2.

SUPPLY TABLE FOR HOSPITALS—Continued.

ARTICLES.	Quantities for one year for commands of				
	From 100 to 200.	From 200 to 300.	From 300 to 400.	500 men.	1 000 men.
Wine, bottles of..........doz..	2	4	6	8	16
BEDDING.					
Bed sacks..................no..	10	20	30	40	80
Bedsteads, iron............no..	6–10	12–20	18–30	24–40	48–80
Blankets, woollen..........no..	10–20	20–40	30–60	40–80	80–160
Coverlets..................no..	10	20	30	40	80
Gutta percha cloth.........yds..	4	6	8	10	16
Mattresses.................no..	2	4	6	8	16
Musquito bars..............no..	6–10	12–20	18–30	24–40	48–80
Pillow cases...............no..	25	50	75	100	200
" ticks....................no..	10	20	30	40	80
Sheets.....................no..	40	80	120	200	400
FURNITURE, DRESSINGS, ETC.					
Bandages, suspensory*......no..	4	8	12	16	32
Binders' boards†...........no..	4	6	8	12	16
Corks, assorted............doz..	12	24	36	48	96
Corkscrews.................no..	1	1	2	2	3
Cotton batting.............lb..	1	2	3	4	8
" wadding..................lb..	1	2	3	4	8
Flannel, red...............yds..	5	10	15	20	40
Funnels, glass.............no..	1	1	2	2	4
" tin......................no..	1	1	2	2	2
Hatchets...................no..	1	1	2	2	2
Hones (in wood)‡...........no..	1	1	1	1	1
Ink powder.................papers..	2	2	3	3	4
Inkstands..................no..	1	1	2	2	2
Linen......................yds..	5	10	15	20	40
Lint.......................lb..	4	6	8	10	20
Measures, graduated........no..	3	3	4	6	6
" tin......................sets..	1	1	1	1	1
Medicine cups and glasses‖.no..	3	6	9	12	24
Mills, coffee..............no..	2	2	2	3	4
Mortars and pestles, glass..no..	1	1	2	2	2
" " " iron...no..	1	1	1	1	1
" " " wedgewood............no..	1	2	2	3	3
Muslin.....................yds..	25	50	75	100	200
Needles, sewing............no..	25	25	25	25	50
Oiled silk or gutta percha tissue, or india-rubber tissue.yds..	4	6	6	8	12

* Assorted. † 18 inches by 4. ‡ inches by 1. ‖ 2 cups to 1 glass.

SUPPLY TABLE FOR HOSPITALS—Continued.

ARTICLES.	Quantities for one year for commands of				
	From 100 to 200.	From 200 to 300.	From 300 to 400.	500 men.	1.000 men.
Pans, bed ....no..	2	2	3	4	5
Paper envelopes* ....no..	100	125	150	200	250
" filtering..........quires..	½	1	2	2	3
" wrapping ....quires..	10	12	15	15	20
" writing† ....quires..	12	20	20	20	30
Pencils, hair .... no..	12	18	24	30	50
" lead ....no..	6	8	10	12	18
Pens, steel ....doz..	2	3	3	4	6
Pill boxes ....papers..	3	6	9	12	24
" machine ....no..	1	1	1	1	1
Pins, assorted..........papers..	2	4	6	8	16
Quills ....no..	25	24	50	50	50
Rain gauges ....no..	1	1	1	1	1
Razors.....................no..	1	1	1	1	2
Razor strops ....no..	1	1	1	1	2
Scales and weights, apothecary's ....sets..	1	1	2	2	2
Scales and weights, shop.. sets..	1	1	1	1	1
Scissors ....no..	2	2	2	3	4
Sheep skins, dressed ....no..	4	6	8	10	12
Silk, surgeons ....oz..	¼	¼	½	½	1
" green ....yds..	½	1	2	2½	5
Spatulas ....no..	3	3	4	6	12
Sponge.................... lb..	½	½	¾	¾	1
Tape‡ ....pieces..	4	8	12	16	32
Thermometers and hygrometers ....no..	2	2	2	2	2
Thermometers ....no..	1	1	1	1	1
Thread, linen... ....oz..	4	4	6	6	8
Tiles.......... ....no..	2	3	3	3	4
Tow.......................lb..	1	2	2	3	5
Towels .... no..	20	30	50	75	150
Twine.....................lb..	1	1	1½	1½	3
Urinals ....no..	2	3	5	6	10
Vials, assorted............doz..	6	12	18	24	48
Wafers (½ oz. boxes)........no..	1	1	2	2	3
Wax, sealing ....sticks..	3	3	4	4	6

* Assorted. 3 sizes—"Official business" printed on each. † Foolscap, letter and note—white; blue ruled. ‡ One quarter, woollen: three quarters, cotton.

If the following articles of Hospital Furniture cannot be obtained with the hospital fund, they may be procured from a quartermaster or medical disbursing officer, by special requisition:

ARTICLES.

Basins, wash.
Bowls.
Brushes.
Buckets.
Candlesticks.
Clothes Lines.
Cups.
Dippers and Ladles.
Graters.
Gridirons.
Kettles, tea.
Knives and Forks.
Lamps and Lanterns.
Locks and Keys.
Mugs.
Pans, frying.
" sauce.
Pitchers.
Plates and Dishes.
Pots, chamber and chair.
" coffee and tea.
Sadirons.
Shovels, fire.
Snuffers.
Spoons.
Tongs and Pokers.
Tumblers.
Woodsaws.

Standard Supply Table for Field Service.

ARTICLES.	QUANTITIES.		
	Reg't 3 mos.	Bat. 3 mos.	Comp. 3 mos.
MEDICINES.			
Acidi acetici .... lb..	1	½	½
" sulph. aromatici .... lb..	1	½	¼
" tannici .... oz..	2	1	1
Ætheris sulphurici loti .... lb..	2	1	1
Alcoholis .... bott..	10	5	3
Aluminis .... lb..	1	½	¼
Ammoniæ carbonatis .... oz..	16	8	4
Antimonii et potass. tartratis .... oz..	2	1	1
Argenti nitratis (crystals) .... oz..	2	1	½
" " (fused) .... oz..	2	1	½
Camphoræ .... lb..	4	2	1
Cerati resinæ .... lb..	2	1	½
" simplicis .... lb..	8	4	2
Chloroformi .... lb..	2	1	1
Copaibæ .... lb..	2	1	½
Creasoti .... oz..	2	1	1
Cupri sulphatis .... oz..	4	2	1
Emplastri adhæsivi .... yds..	10	5	3
" cantharidis .... lb..	4	2	1
" ichthyocollæ .... yds..	10	5	3
Extracti belladonnæ .... oz..	1	1	1
" colchici acetici .... oz..	2	1	1
" colocynthidis comp .... oz..	16	8	4
" glycyrrhizæ .... lb..	2	1	½
Hydrargyri chloridi corrosivi .... oz..	½	½	½
" " mitis .... lb..	2	1	½
Iodinii .... oz..	4	2	1
Liquoris Ammoniæ .... lb..	4	2	1
" potass. arsenitis .... oz..	4	2	1
Magnesiæ sulphatis .... lb..	20	10	5
Massæ pil: hydrargyri .... oz..	16	8	4
Morphiæ sulphatis .... dr..	4	2	1
Olei caryophylli .... oz..	1	1	1
" menthæ piperitæ .... oz..	2	1	1
" olivæ .... bott..	8	4	2
" ricini .... qt. bott..	12	6	3
" terebinthinæ .... qt. bott..	8	4	2
" tiglii .... dr..	2	1	1
Pilul: cathartic: comp: (U. S.) ...... doz..	8	4	2
" opii (U. S.) .... doz..	8	4	2
" quiniæ sulphatis (3 grs.) .... doz..	8	4	2
Plumbi acetatis .... lb..	2	1	½
Potassæ bicarbonatis .... lb..	1	½	¼
" chloratis .... lb..	2	1	½
" nitratis .... lb..	1	½	¼

SUPPLY TABLE FOR FIELD SERVICE—Continued.

ARTICLES.	QUANTITIES.		
	Reg't 3 mos.	Bat. 3 mos.	Comp. 3 mos.
Potassii iodidi....................oz..	8	4	2
Pulveris acaciæ....................lb..	4	2	1
" capsici....................lb..	½	¼	¼
" ferri per sulphatis....................oz..	4	2	1
" ipecacuanhæ....................lb..	1	½	¼
" " et opii....................oz..	8	4	4
" lini....................lb..	16	8	4
" opii....................lb..	2	1	½
" rhei....................lb..	½	¼	¼
" sinapis nigræ....................lb..	12	6	3
Quiniæ sulphatis....................oz..	24	12	6
Sacchari....................lb..	10	5	2
Saponis....................lb..	8	4	2
Sodæ bicarbonatis....................lb..	1	½	¼
Spiritus ammoniæ aromatici....................oz..	4	2	2
" ætheris nitrici....................lb..	2	1	½
" vini gallici....................bott..	24	12	6
Tincturæ ferri chloridi....................lb..	1	½	¼
" opii....................oz..	16	8	6
Unguenti hydrargyri....................lb..	1	½	¼
" " nitratis....................lb..	½	¼	¼
Zinci acetatis....................oz..	2	1	1
" sulphatis....................oz..	2	1	1
" chlorid....................oz..	1	½	½
INSTRUMENTS.			
* A case of instruments for general operations, containing all instruments necessary for amputations, resections and trephining.			
* A pocket case, containing all instruments required in the daily routine of surgical dressings.			
* A case of assorted catheters.			
Buck's spongeholder for the throat....................no..	1	1	1
Cupping glasses and tins†....................no..	16	8	4
Lancets, spring....................no..	1	1	1
" thumb (with cases)....................no..	6	4	2
Pocket....................sets..	1	1	1
Probangs, whalebone....................no..	12	6	2
Scarificators....................no..	4	2	1
Splints (major)....................sets..	1	1	1

*These are instruments which a field surgeon cannot do without, and have, apparently, been accidentally omitted from the supply table of the Confederate service.

†Half glass, half tin.

SUPPLY TABLE FOR FIELD SERVICE—Continued.

ARTICLES.	QUANTITIES.		
	Reg't 3 mos.	Bat. 3 mos.	Comp. 3 mos.
Syringes, enema*......no..	4	2	1
" penis, glass......no..	8	4	2
" " india-rubber......no..	8	4	2
Teeth extracting......sets..	1	1	1
Tongue depressor (hinge)......no..	1	1	1
Tourniquets, field......no..	8	4	2
" spiral......no..	2	2	1
Trusses, hernia......no..	6	3	2
BOOKS.			
Anatomy (surgical)......cop..	1	1	1
Medical Practice......cop..	1	1	1
Regulations for medical department......cop..	1	1	1
Surgery (operative)......cop..	1	1	1
Thompson's Conspectus......cop..	1	1	1
Blank......no..	4	4	4
HOSPITAL STORES.			
Arrowroot......lb..	10	5	3
Candles (sperm)......lb..	2	1	1
Farina......lb..	10	5	3
Ginger, (fluid extract)......lb..	1	½	¼
Nutmegs......oz..	8	4	2
Tea......lb..	30	15	7
Whiskey, bottles of......doz..	2	1	½
BEDDING.			
Blankets, woollen (brown)......no..	20–40	10–20	10
Blanket cases (of canvas, after pattern)...no..	1 for	10 bla	nkets
Gutta percha cloth......yds..	8	4	2
" " bed covers†......no..	8	4	2
Musquito bars......no..	12	6	4
FURNITURE AND DRESSINGS.			
Bandages,‡ roller, assorted......doz..	14	7	4

*1 Davidson's; 1 hard rubber, 6 oz.

†So constructed, as to form, when united a continuous spread or covering.

‡1 dozen, 1 inch wide, 1 yard long.
2 " 2 " 3 "
2 " 2½ " 3 "
1 " 3 " 4 "
½ " 3½ " 5 "
½ " 4 " 6 "

SUPPLY TABLE FOR FIELD SERVICE—Continued.

ARTICLES.	QUANTITIES.		
	Reg't 3 mos.	Bat. 3 mos.	Comp. 3 mos.
Bandages, suspensory, assorted ....no..	12	6	4
Binders' boards (18 inches by 4)..........no..	18	9	5
Buckets, leather.........................no..	4	2	2
Corks, assorted........................doz..	12	6	3
Corkscrews ....no..	2	1	1
Cotton batting...........................lb..	2	1	½
" wadding ....lb..	2	1	½
Flannel (red) ....yds..	5	3	2
Hatchets ....no..	2	1	1
Hones (4 inches by 1, in wood)............no..	1	1	1
Ink, 2-ounce bottles.....................no..	12	6	3
Knapsacks, hospital*.....................no..			
Lanterns ....no..	4	2	1
Lint.....................................lb..	8	4	2
Litters and stretchers, hand*.............no..			
" horse*.........................no..			
Measures, graduated, assorted†...........no..	4	2	2
Medicine chests ....no..			
" cups and glasses‡ ....no..	6	3	2
" panniers.......................no..			
Mess chests (see note)...................no..			
Mills, coffee............................no..	2	1	1
Mortars and pestles, Wedgewood (small)...no..	2	1	1
Muslin ....yds..	20	10	5
Needles, sewing (assorted, in a case) ......no..	25	25	25
Oiled silk or gutta percha tissue, or india-rubber tissue.........................yds..	8	4	2
Pans, bed‖...............................no..	2	1	1
Paper envelopes, assorted§...............no..	100	50	25
Paper, wrapping ....quires..	6	3	1
" writing¶.......................quires..	12	6	3
Pencils, hair ....no..	24	12	6
" lead (of Faber's make, No. 2).....no..	12	6	3
Pens, steel.............................doz..	4	2	1
Pill boxes (wood)....................papers..	2	1	1
" (tin) ....no..	6	6	6
Pins, assorted (large and medium).....papers..	4	2	2
Razors ....no..	1	1	1
Razor strops.............................no..	1	1	1

* According to pattern.

† 6 oz., 2 oz., minim.

‡ 2 cups to 1 glass.

‖ Of hard india-rubber or other material. Shovel.

§ 50 letter, 25 note, 25 large. "Official Business" printed on each.

¶ 2 foolscap, 6 letter, 4 note, white; blue ruled.

SUPPLY TABLE FOR FIELD SERVICE—Continued.

ARTICLES.	QUANTITIES.		
	Reg't 3 mos.	Bat. 3 mos.	Comp. 3 mos.
Scales and weights, apothecary's.........sets..	1	1	1
Scissors ....no..	4	2	2
Sheep skins, dressed....................no..	4	2	1
Silk, surgeons' ....oz..	½	¼	¼
" green ....yds..	1	½	½
Spatulas.................................no..	6	3	2
Sponge (washed).......................lb..	1	½	¼
Tape ....pieces..	4	2	1
Thread, linen...........................oz..	2	1	1
Tiles.....................................no..	2	1	1
Towels ....no..	40	20	10
Twine ....lb..	½	¼	¼
Urinals...................................no..	4	2	1
Vials, assorted (1 oz. and 2 oz.) ....doz..	4	2	1
Wafers (½ ounce boxes) ....no..	1	1	1
Wax, sealing.......................sticks..	2	1	1

NOTE TO PRECEDING TABLE.

FURNITURE OF MESS CHEST.

8 Basins, tin.
2 Boxes, pepper and salt.
6 Cups, tin.
4 Canisters (for tea, coffee, sugar and butter).
2 Dippers and ladles.
1 Grater.
1 Gridiron.
1 Kettle, tea, iron.
12 Knives and forks.
6 Mugs (Britannia, half-pint).
1 Pan, frying.
1 Pan, sauce.
8 Plates (6) and dishes (2), tin.
1 Pot, iron.
2 Pots, coffee and tea, tin.
12 Spoons, iron [table (6) and tea (6)].
1 Tray, tin.
6 Tumblers, tin.

The Standard Supply Tables contain all the articles to be purchased by medical purveyors, except on the orders of the Surgeon-General; but any less quantity may be required or any article omitted at the discretion of the medical officer.

FORM 1.

REPORT OF THE SICK AND WOUNDED AT , FOR THE ENDING 18—.

GENERAL SUMMARY.

Total.

Rate per

FORM 1—Continued.

DISCHARGES ON SURGEON'S CERTIFICATE, AND DEATHS.

Name.		Rank.	Regiment.	Company.	Disease.	Date of discharge from service.	Date of death.
Surname.	Christian name.						

REMARKS.

NOTES.—Discharges on Surgeon's certificate, and deaths occurring among those of the command *not* on sick report, will be also reported, but separated from the others by a double line drawn across the page. The remarks will in each case specify the manner in which the disease originated, when it is known.

In every case of the death of an officer, whether on duty or not, a special report is to be made to the Surgeon-General.

FORM 1—Continued.

ENDORSEMENT.

REPORT OF SICK AND WOUNDED.

FOR THE

Quarter ending 186 ,

Station:

SURGEON.

COMMAND.

REGIMENTS.	COMPANIES.

FORM 2.

Return of the Medical Officers of the Regular Army, Volunteer Corps, and Militia, including Physicians employed under contract, serving in the Department of ——, for the Month of ——, 186—.*

No.	NAMES.	RANK.	POST OR STATION.	WITH WHAT TROOPS SERVING.	REMARKS.

Surgeon.

NOTE.—The names will be arranged in the following order: 1st. Medical Officers of the Regular Army; 2d. Those of Volunteer Corps and Militia; 3d. Private Physicians. In the column of "Remarks." will be noted all changes in the position of Medical Officers and Private Physicians, whether on duty, or on leave of absence; giving the number, date and source of the order directing or authorizing such change, the time of the departure of the officers from their posts, and the date of their return to duty. If to a new post, its position must be indicated by reference to some known point, as —— miles north from —— river, town, or post-office. The remarks opposite the names of Private Physicians, will state, in addition to the above, the name and rank of the party making the contract, the date thereof, the monthly compensation, and the date of their discharge from service.

The Medical Directors will require from the Medical Officers and Private Physicians in their respective Departments, monthly reports to enable them to make out and transmit this Return to the Surgeon-General.

FORM 3.

RETURN OF MEDICAL AND HOSPITAL PROPERTY.

ARTICLES AND CHARACTERS OR QUANTITIES.	On hand at last return.	Received since last return.	Total.	Expended with the sick.	Issued.	Lost or destroyed by unavoidable accident.	Worn out, or unfit for use.	Total expended, etc.	On hand.	REMARKS.

I certify, on honor, that the above return is correct, to the best of my knowledge, and that the medicines and stores have been expended with the sick belonging to the army alone.

——— ———, *Surgeon.*

N. B.—Returns will always be transmitted in duplicate, and by different mails.

FORM 4.

Abstract of Medical and Hospital Property received and issued at ——, in the quarter ending on the —— day of ——, 186 , by —— ——, Medical Purveyor.

ARTICLES AND CHARACTERS OR QUANTITIES.	RECEIVED.						ISSUED.								
	Vou. No. 1.	Vou. No. 2.	Vou. No. 3.	Vou. No. 4.	Vou. No. 5.	Total.	Vou. No. 1.	Vou. No. 2.	Vou. No. 3.	Vou. No. 4.	Vou. No. 5.	Vou. No. 6.	Vou. No. 7.	Vou. No. 8.	Total.

I certify that the above abstract is correct.

—— ——, *Medical Purveyor.*

N. B.—Invoices and receipts must accompany this abstract.

FORM 5.

REQUISITION FOR MEDICAL AND HOSPITAL SUPPLIES.

Station: ——. Period: ——.

From —— to ——.

Command: Officers, ——; Enlisted Men, ——; All others entitled to Medicines, ——; Total, ——.

ARTICLES AND CHARACTERS OR QUANTITIES.	On hand.	Wanted.	ARTICLES AND CHARACTERS OR QUANTITIES.	On hand.	Wanted.
Acaciæ. - - - - - lb.					
Acidi acetici, - - - lb.					
" arseniosi, - - - oz.					

Date: ——

—— ——,
Surgeon.

N. B.—Requisitions will exhibit the quantity of each and every article "on hand," whether more wanted or not. They will be transmitted in duplicate, and by different mails.

Form 6.

SPECIAL REQUISITION FOR SUPPLIES OF MEDICINES, Etc.

Requisition for Medicines (Hospital Stores, etc.) required at ———, for ———.

Acet: plumbi, lb. i.
Pulv: cinchonæ, lbs. x.
Etc., etc.
Etc., etc.

I certify that the medicines above required are necessary for the sick at ———, in consequence of [here state whether from loss, damage, etc., etc.], and that the requisition is agreeable to the Supply Table.

——— ———, *Surgeon.*

Approved:

——— ———, *Commanding Officer.*

Received, ——— 186—, of ——— ———, the articles above enumerated.

——— ———, *Surgeon.*

Form 7.

ACCOUNT FOR MEDICINES, ETC., PURCHASED BY A SURGEON OR AN OFFICER OF THE QUARTERMASTER'S DEPARTMENT.

THE CONFEDERATE STATES,

To A B, Dr.

Acet: plumb; lb; i, at 50 cts.	$ 50
Pulv: cinchon: lbs: x, at $2	20 00
Etc., etc., etc.	

I certify that the articles above charged, for the use of the sick at ——, are agreeable to the foregoing requisition, and that the charges are reasonable and just.

—— ——, *Surgeon.*

Received, —— 186—, of —— ——, —— dollars and —— cents, in full of the above account.

A. B.

NOTE.—The above certificate may be signed by the Surgeon making the requisition, or by any Surgeon or Assistant Surgeon belonging to the army.

FORM 8.

ACCOUNT OF HOSPITAL STORES, FURNITURE, ETC., ISSUED.

DATE.	Rice.	Sugar.	Tea.	Wine.	Brandy.	Coffee.	Etc.	Etc.	Etc.			REMARKS.
	Lbs.	Lbs.	Oz.	Qts.	Qts.	Lbs.	Etc.	Etc.	Etc.			

Form 9.

ACCOUNT OF CLOTHING, ARMS, EQUIPMENTS, Etc., OF PATIENTS IN HOSPITAL.

Date.	No.	Names.	Rank.	Regiment or corps.	Company.	Coats.	Jackets.	Overalls.	Etc.	Muskets.	Knapsacks.	Etc.	Etc.	Etc.				When delivered.	Remarks.
																			The remarks will note to whom the articles were delivered; what money, etc. were left by those who die, and to whom they were given.

FORM 10.

ACCOUNT OF FURNITURE, COOKING UTENSILS, BEDDING, etc., IN USE.

No. of ward or kitchen.	Bunks.	Bed sacks.	Sheets.	Blankets.	Kettles.	Spoons.	Knives.	Forks.	Etc.	Etc.										Lost.	Worn out.	Destroyed by order.	Returned to steward.	REMARKS.
																								The remarks will state how articles have been lost, and by whom destroyed, or the persons suspected, etc.

FORM 11.

REGISTER.

NAMES.	Rank.	Regiment or corps.	Company.	COMPLAINT.	Admitted.	Returned to duty.	Deserted.	Discharged from service.	Sent to general hospital.	On furlough.	Died.	REMARKS.

N. B.—Both christian and surname will be registered.

FORM 12.

PRESCRIPTION BOOK, DIET BOOK, AND DIET TABLE.

NAMES.	Sunday.	Monday.	Tuesday.	Wednesday.	Thursday.	Friday.	Saturday.

The spaces in the Prescription Book are to be filled up with the prescriptions at length, the times of administering the medicines and the quantities to be given at each time. The diet of the patients will be divided into full, half, and low, to be designated in the Diet Book by the letters F. H. and L.; and in order that the steward may have precise instructions for delivering the hospital stores, etc., the surgeon will, from time to time, insert in the Diet Book written directions of the quantity of each article in his store room which he may think necessary to each degree of diet. To each ten patients, for example, on low diet, a certain quantity of tea, sugar, etc. To each ten on half diet, a certain quantity of rice, milk, etc. These proportions will soon become familiar to the steward, who has only to refer to the letters in the Diet Book, to ascertain the whole quantity of any article to be delivered for the day, as well as the quantity for each ward. When any liquor is directed, or any other article not contained in these general instructions of the surgeon, the precise quantity directed for each patient will be noted in the Diet Book. The Diet Tables are to be filled up daily from the Diet Book, and hung up in each ward of a general hospital.

FORM 13.

ARMY OF THE CONFEDERATE STATES.

(Coat of Arms.)

Certificate of Disability for Discharge.

A B, of Captain ———'s company, (—), of the —— regiment of Confederate States ———, was enlisted by —— ——, of the —— regiment of ——, at ———, on the —— day of ———, to serve —— years; he was born in ———, in the State of ———, is —— years of age, —— feet —— inches high, —— complexion, —— eyes, —— hair, and by occupation, when enlisted, ———. During the last two months said soldier has been unfit for duty —— days.

(The company commander will here add a statement of all the *facts* known to him concerning the disease or wound, or cause of disability of the soldier; the time, place, manner, and all the circumstances under which the injury occurred, or disease originated or appeared; the duty or service or situation of the soldier at the time the injury was received or disease contracted, or supposed to be contracted; and whatever facts may aid a judgment as to the cause, immediate or remote, of the disability and the circumstances attending it.)

C D, *Commanding Company.*

(When the *facts* are not known to the company commander, the certificate of any officer, or affidavit of other person having such knowledge, will be appended.)

I CERTIFY that I have carefully examined the said ——— of Captain ———'s company, and find him incapable of performing the duties of a soldier because of (here describe particularly the disability, wound, or disease; the extent to which it deprives him of the use of any limb or faculty, or affects his health, strength, activity, constitution, or capacity to labor or earn his subsistence). The Surgeon will add, from his knowledge of the facts and circumstances, and from the evidence in the case, his professional opinion of the cause or origin of the disability.

E F, *Surgeon.*

(DUPLICATES).

NOTES.—1. When a *probable* case for *pension, special care* must be taken to state the *degree* of disability.

2 The *place* where the *soldier* desires to be *addressed* may be here added

Town— *County*— *State*—

Form 14.

MORNING REPORT OF THE SURGEON OF A REGIMENT, POST, OR GARRISON.

Date.	Company.	Remaining at last report.		Taken sick.	Total.		Returned to duty.	Discharged.	Sent to general hospital.	Died.	Remaining.		Remarks.
		In hospital.	In quarters.		In hospital.	In quarters.					In hospital.	In quarters.	

FORM 15.

CONTRACT WITH A PRIVATE PHYSICIAN.

This contract, entered into this —— day of ——, 18—, at ——, State of ——, between —— ——, of the C. S. Army, and Dr. —— ——, of ——, in the State of ——, witnesseth, that for the consideration hereafter mentioned, the said Dr. —— —— promises and agrees to perform the duties of a medical officer, agreeably to the Army Regulations, at —— (*and to furnish the necessary medicines*). And the said —— —— promises and agrees, on behalf of the Confederate States, to pay, or cause to be paid, to the said Dr. ——, the sum of —— dollars for each and every month he shall continue to perform the services above stated, which shall be his full compensation, and in lieu of all allowances and emoluments whatsoever (*except that for medicines furnished, which shall be at the rate of —— per cent. on his monthly pay, to be determined by the Surgeon-General*). This contract to continue till determined by the said doctor, or the commanding officer for the time being, or the Surgeon-General.

[SEAL.]

Signed, sealed, and delivered, } in presence of— }

[SEAL.]

I certify that the number of persons entitled to medical attendance, agreeably to regulations, at —— is ——, and that no competent physician can be obtained at a lower rate.

—— ——, *Commanding Officer.*

FORM 16.

A Monthly Statement of the Hospital Fund at ——, for the month of ——, 186—.

DR.				
To balance due hospital last month, - - - -				$ 0 00
1,532 rations, being whole amount due this month, at 9½ cents per ration, - - - -				145 54
ISSUED.				
CR.				
By the following provisions, at contract prices:				
283½	lbs. of pork, at 6 cents per pound,		$17 01	
690	lbs. of fresh beef, at 4c. per pound,		27 60	
1,612 2/16	lbs. of flour, at 2 cents per pound,		32 24¼	
10	lbs. of hard bread, at 3½c. per lb.		0 35	
70	lbs. of rice, at 6 cents per pound,		4 20	
56	lbs. of coffee, at 9 cts. per pound,		5 04	
193 14/16	lbs. of sugar, at 8 cts. per pound,		15 51	
17⅛	qrts. of vinegar, at 5c. per quart,		0 85⅝	
15 5/16	lbs. of candles, at 12c. per pound,		1 83¾	
61¼	lbs. of soap, at 6 cents per pound,		3 67½	
16⅞	qrts. of salt, at 3 cents per quart,		0 50⅝	
12	galls. molasses, at 28c. per gallon,		3 36	
			$112 18¾	
PURCHASED.				
2 prs. of chickens, at 87½c. per pair, - - - - -		$1 75		
4 qts. of milk, at 7c. per quart,		0 28		
3 doz. oranges, at 25c. per doz.		0 75	2 78	
Total expended, -		–	–	114 96¾
Balance due this month,		–	–	$30 57¼

—— ——, *Surgeon.*

[Date.]

Form 17.

FORM OF A MEDICAL CERTIFICATE,

FOR LEAVE OF ABSENCE.

—— —— of the —— regiment of ———, having applied for a certificate on which to ground an application for leave of absence, I do hereby certify that I have carefully examined this officer, and find that ———. [Here the nature of the disease, wound, or disability, is to be fully stated, and the period during which the officer has suffered under its effects.] And that, in consequence thereof, he is, in my opinion, unfit for duty. I further declare my belief that he will not be able to resume his duties in a period less than ———. [Here state candidly and explicitly the opinion as to the period which will probably elapse before the officer will be able to resume his duties. When there is no reason to expect a recovery, or when the prospect of recovery is distant and uncertain, it must be so stated.]

Dated ———, this —— day of ———.

Signature of the Medical officer. } —— ———.

Form 18.

RECORD OF RECRUITS EXAMINED BY —— ——, AT ——.

Date.	Name.	Where Born.		Age.	Profession.	By whom enlisted.	Remarks.
		Town or County.	State or Kingdom.				

EXTRACTS

FROM THE

REGULATIONS FOR THE UNITED STATES ARMY.

(EDITION OF 1857.)

QUARTERMASTER'S DEPARTMENT.

715..Provides "that soldiers be not permitted to leave the ranks to assist the wounded, unless by express permission, which is only to be given after the action is decided. The highest interest and duty is to win the victory, which only can insure proper care of the wounded."

716.."Before an action, the Quartermaster of the division makes all the necessary arrangements for the transportation of the wounded. He establishes the ambulance depôts in the rear, and gives his assistants the necessary instruction for the service of the ambulance wagons, and other means of removing the wounded."

717.."The ambulance depôt, to which the wounded are carried or directed for immediate treatment, is generally established at the most convenient building nearest the field of battle. A *red flag* marks its place, or the way to it, to the conductors of the ambulance, and to the wounded who can walk."

718.."The active ambulance follows the troop engaged to succor the wounded and remove them to the depôt. For this purpose, the conductor should always have the necessary assistants that the soldiers may have no excuse for leaving the ranks for that object."

719..The medical director of the division, after consultation with the Quartermaster-General, distributes the medical officers and hospital attendants, at his disposal, to the depôts and active ambulances. He will send officers and attendants, when practicable, to the active ambulances, to relieve the wounded who require treatment before being removed from the ground. He will see that the depôts and ambulances are provided with the necessary apparatus, medicines and stores. He will take post and render his professional services at the principal depôt.

720..If the enemy endangers the depôt, the Quartermaster takes the orders of the General to remove it, or to strengthen its guard.

721..The wounded in the depôts, and the sick, are removed, as soon as possible, to the hospitals that have been established by the Quartermaster-General of the Army, on the flanks or rear of the army.

782..In sieges, the field officer of the trenches sees that men and litters are always ready to bring off the wounded.

929..No officer making returns of property shall drop from his return any public property as worn out or unserviceable until it has been condemned, after proper inspection, and ordered to be so dropped.

935...Every officer having public money to account for, and failing to render his account thereof quarter-yearly, with the vouchers necessary to its correct and prompt settlement, within three months after the expiration of the quarter, if resident in the United States, and within six months if resident in a foreign country, will be promptly dismissed by the President, unless he shall explain the default to the satisfaction of the President. (Act January 31, 1823.)

936..Every officer entrusted with public money or property shall render all prescribed returns and accounts to the bureau of the department in which he is serving, where all such returns and accounts shall pass through a rigid administrative scrutiny before the money accounts are transmitted to the proper offices of the Treasury Department for settlement.

991...The sick will be transported on the application of the medical officers to the Quartermaster.

1005..Assistant surgeons, approved by an examining board and commissioned, receive transportation in the execution of their first order to duty.

1013..The allowance and change of straw for the sick is regulated by the surgeons.

1013. . Officers receiving clothing or camp and garrison equipage, will render quarterly returns of it to the Quartermaster-General.

1073. . Issues to the hospital will be on returns by the medical officer, for such provisions only as are actually required for the sick and the attendants. The cost of such parts of the ration as are issued will be charged to the hospital at contract or cost prices, and the hospital will be credited by the whole number of complete rations due through the month at contract or cost prices (see Note 7); the balance, constituting the *Hospital Fund*, or any portion of it, may be expended by the commissary, on the requisition of the medical officer, in the purchase of any article for the subsistence or comfort of the sick, not authorized to be otherwise furnished (see Form 3). At large depôts or general hospitals, this fund may be partly expended for the benefit of dependent posts or detachments, on requisitions approved by the medical director or senior surgeon of the district.

1074. . The articles purchased for the hospital, as well as those issued from the subsistence storehouse, will be included in the surgeon's certificate of issues to the hospital, and borne on the monthly return of provisions received and issued. Vouchers for purchases for the hospital must either be certified by the surgeon or accompanied by his requisition.

1075. . Abstracts of the issues to the hospital will be made by the commissary, certified by the surgeon and countersigned by the commanding officer.

1079. . An extra issue of fifteen pounds of tallow or ten of sperm candles, per month, may be made to the principal guard of each camp and garrison, on the order of the commanding officer. Extra issues of soap, candles, and vinegar, are permitted to the hospital when the surgeon does not avail himself of the commutation of the hospital rations, or when there is no hospital fund; salt, in small quantities, may be issued for public horses and cattle. When the officers of the medical department find anti-scorbutics necessary for the health of the troops, the commanding officer may order issues of fresh vegetables, pickled onions, sour-crout, or molasses, with an extra quantity of rice and vinegar. (Potatoes are usually issued at the rate of one pound per ration, and onions at the rate of three bushels in lieu of one of beans.) Occasional issues (extra) of molasses are made—two quarts to one hundred rations—and of dried apples of from one to one and a half bushels to one hundred rations. Troops at sea are recommended to draw rice and an extra issue of molasses in lieu of beans. When anti-scorbutics are issued, the medical officer will certify the necessity, and the circumstances which cause it, upon the abstract of extra issues.

EXTRACTS FROM GENERAL ORDERS.

I. Ambulances will not be used for any other than the specific purpose for which they are designed, viz: the transportation of the sick and wounded; and those hereafter provided for the army will be made according to a pattern to be furnished the quartermaster's department by the Surgeon-General.

II. Paragraph 963 of the Regulations for the Army is so far amended as to allow the medical director and medical purveyor of a military department one room each as an office; and fuel therefor from the 1st of October to the 30th of April, at the rate of one cord of wood per month.

* * * * * * *

Officers of the medical department may, by virtue of their commissions, command all enlisted men, like other commissioned officers. Paragraph 13, Army Regulations, will not be interpreted to restrict that authority.

* * * * * * *

---

1. Boards of Survey will not be resorted to for the *condemnation* of public property, but only to establish data by which

questions of administrative responsibility may be determined, and the adjustment of accounts facilitated: such as to assess the damage which public property has sustained from any extraordinary cause, not ordinary wear, either in transit or in store, or in actual use, and to set forth the circumstances and fix the responsibility of such damage, whether on the carrier, or the person accountable for the property or having it immediately in charge; to report from examination the circumstances and amount of the loss or deficiency of public property by accident, unusual wastage, or otherwise, and fix the responsibility of such loss or deficiency; to make inventories of property ordered to be abandoned, when the articles have not been enumerated in the orders; to assess the prices at which damaged clothing may be issued to troops, and the proportion in which supplies shall be issued in consequence of damage that renders them at the usual rate unequal to the allowance which the regulations contemplate; to verify the discrepancy between the invoices and the actual quantity or description of property transferred from one officer to another, and ascertain, as far as possible, where and how the discrepany has occurred, whether in the hands of the carrier or the officer making the transfer; and to make inventories and report on the condition of public property in the possession of officers at the time of their death. The action of the Board for the authorized object will be complete with the approval of the commanding officer, but liable to revision by higher authority. In no case, however, will the report of the Board supersede the depositions which the law requires with reference to deficiencies and damage.

2. Boards of Survey will not be convened by any other than the commanding officer present, and will be composed of as many officers, not exceeding three, as may be present for duty, the commanding officer and the officer responsible in the matter to be reported on being excluded; but in case the two latter only are present, then the one not responsible will perform the duties, and the responsible officer will perform them if no other officer is present. The proceedings of the Board will be signed by each member, and a copy forwarded by the approving officer to the head-quarters of the department or army in the field, as

the case may be, duplicates being furnished to the officer accountable for the property.

3..All surveys and reports having in view the *condemnation* of public property, for whatever cause, will be made by the commanding officers of posts or other separate commands, or by inspectors-general, or inspectors specially designated by the commander of a department or an army in the field, or by higher authority. Such surveys and reports having a different object from those of Boards of Survey, will be required independently of any action of a Board on the same property.

4..When public property is received by any officer, he will make a careful examination to ascertain its quality and condition, but without breaking packages until issues are to be made, unless there is cause to suppose the contents defective; and in any of the cases supposed in the first paragraph, he will apply for a Board of Survey for the purposes therein set forth. If he deem the property unfit for use, and that the public interest requires it to be condemned, he will, in addition, report the fact for that purpose to the commanding officer, who will make a critical inspection, or cause it to be made by an inspector-general or special inspector, according to the nature of his command. If the inspector deem the property fit, it shall be received and used. If not, he will forward a formal inspection report to the commander empowered to give orders in the case. The same rule will be observed, according to the nature of the case, with reference to property already on hand. The person accountable for the property, or having it in charge, will submit an inventory, which will accompany or be embodied in the inspection report, stating how long the property has been in his possession, how long in use, and from whom it was received. The inspector's report will state the exact condition of each article, and what disposition it is expedient to make of it: as, to be destroyed, to be dropped as being of no value, to be broken up, to be repacked or repaired, or to be sold. The inspector will certify on his report that he has examined each article, and that its condition is as stated. If the commanding officer, who ordinarily would be the inspector, is himself accountable for the property, the next officer in rank present for duty will act as the inspector. The authority of inspection and condemnation will not, without special instructions, extend to commanding officers of arsenals with reference to ordnance and ordnance stores, but may in regard to other unserviceable supplies.

5. . An officer commanding a department or an army in the field, may give orders, on the report of the authorized inspectors, either to sell, destroy, or make such other disposition of condemned property as the case may require, excepting with reference to the sale of ordnance and ordnance stores; but if the property be of very considerable value, and there is reason to suppose that it could be advantageously applied or disposed of elsewhere than within his command, he will refer the matter to the chief of the staff department to which it belongs. No other persons than those designated, or the General-in-Chief, will order the final disposition of condemned property, excepting in the case of ordnance and ordnance stores, which are to be dropped or broken up; horses which should be killed to prevent contagion, and provisions or other stores which are deteriorating so rapidly as to require immediate action. In this last case, the inspector may order the destruction or sale of the stores, and, in the other cases, he may direct the dispositions above indicated with reference to them. The inventories will be made in duplicate: one to be retained by the person accountable, and the other to accompany his accounts. When the action of the inspector has been final, a copy of the inventory will be forwarded through the department, or other superior head-quarters, to the chief of the staff department to which the property belongs. When the action of the department or other superior commander is required, the original inventories will be sent to the head-quarters, and returned with the final orders thereon to the person accountable for the property, and a copy of the inventory and orders will be forwarded from the department or other superior head-quarters to the chief of the staff department to which they relate.

6. . Every inspector, member of a Board of Survey, and commander acting on their proceedings, shall be answerable that his action has been proper and judicious, according to the regulations and the circumstances of the case.

7..As far as practicable, every officer in charge of public property, whether it be in use or in store, will endeavor, by timely repairs, to keep it in serviceable condition, for which purpose the necessary means will be allowed on satisfactory requisitions; and property in store so repaired will be issued for further use. Unserviceable arms will be sent to an arsenal for repair, before accumulating in excess of the surplus arms in the company. Provisions and other perishable stores will be repacked whenever it may be necessary for their preservation, and their value will justify the expense, which will be a legitimate charge against the department to which they belong. Public animals will not be condemned for temporary disease or want of condition, but may, by order of the commanding officer, after inspection, be turned in for rest and treatment, if unfit for service for which they are immediately required.

8..Public property shall not be transferred gratuitously from one staff department to another; but when offered for sale, and required for the public service in another staff department in which its use is allowed by regulations, it may be bid in on the order of the commanding officer, or purchased at a fair valuation, to be determined by a Board of Survey, if there should be no other bidder.

9..Paragraph 926, Army Regulations, and so much of any previous orders or regulations as conflicts with the foregoing, are rescinded.

It is desirable to furnish ambulance transportation for forty men per one thousand—twenty lying extended and twenty sitting.

Both two and four wheeled ambulances are desirable for the hospital service.

A two wheeled ambulance is the best for the conveyance of dangerously sick or dangerously wounded men.

It is recommended that the following schedule of transports for the sick and wounded, and for hospital supplies, be adopted for a state of war with a civilized enemy:

For commands of less than three companies, one two wheeled

transport cart for hospital supplies, and to each company one two wheeled ambulance.

For commands of more than three and less than five companies, two two wheeled transport carts, and to each company one two wheeled ambulance.

For a battalion of five companies, one four wheeled ambulance, five two wheeled ambulances, and two two wheeled transport carts. For each additional company less than ten, one two wheeled transport cart.

For a regiment, two four wheeled ambulances, ten two wheeled ambulances, and four two wheeled transport carts.

The transport carts to be made after the models of the two wheeled ambulances (their interior arrangement for the sick excepted), and to have solid board flooring to the body.

It is recommended that in future hospital tents be made according to the pattern of the present tent and of the same material, but smaller, and having on one end a lapel so as to admit of two or more tents being joined and thrown into one with a continuous covering or roof.

The dimensions to be these: In length, fourteen feet; in width, fifteen feet; in height (centre), eleven feet, with a wall four and a half feet, and a "fly" of appropriate size. The ridge pole to be made in two sections after the present pattern, and to measure fourteen feet when joined.

It is contemplated that such a tent will accommodate from eight to ten patients comfortably.

The following allowance of tents for the sick, their attendants, and hospital supplies is recommended:

COMMANDS.	Hospital tents.	Sibley tents.	Common tents.
For one company........	–	1	1
For three companies	1	1	1
For five companies.......	2	1	1
For seven companies	2	1	1
For ten companies	3	1	1

The adoption of a hospital knapsack is recommended to be

carried by a hospital orderly upon the march or in battle, who is habitually to follow the medical officer. The knapsack to be made of light wood; to be divided into four compartments or drawers, and to be covered with canvas. The purpose of this knapsack is to carry, in an accessible shape, such instruments, dressings and medicines as may be needed in an emergency on the march or in the field. The dimensions of the hospital knapsack to be those of the ordinary knapsack.

CORRESPONDENCE.

The Surgeon-General directs that official *letters*, addressed to him by medical officers of the army, be written on letter paper (quarto post) whenever practicable, and not on note or foolscap paper. Also, that the letter be folded in three equal folds parallel with the writing, and endorsed on that fold which corresponds with the top of the sheet; thus:

(Name and rank of writer.)

(Post or station and date of letter.)

(Analysis of contents.)

Appendix No. 2.

MEMORANDUM

FOR THE

INFORMATION OF MEDICAL OFFICERS

IN THE ENGLISH ARMY,

ON TAKING THE FIELD FOR ACTIVE SERVICE.

1. . . . The ambulance equipment for one division of the army, consisting of two brigades of three battalions each—the battalions being 800 strong, should consist of two large store wagons, to be under the care of a purveyor's clerk, at the head-quarters of the division. These wagons to contain a reserve supply of medicines, materials, medical comforts, tents and bedding. Each battalion surgeon should have a pack-horse for the conveyance of his instruments, a few medical comforts for immediate use; such as a bottle of brandy, half pound of tea, one pound of sugar, and four ounces of arrowroot, a few tins of essence of beef, some medicines, and a supply of surgical materials agreeably to the printed scale laid down in the regulations. A spring wagon should also be attached to each battalion for the removal of the wounded off the field, and for the conveyance of the hospital canteens, A and B, with twelve sets of bedding, ten canvas bearers, and the hospital marquee on the line of march: or, when the spring wagons are either small, or required for the

conveyance of sick and wounded, a reserve wagon might be attached to each brigade for the carriage of these articles.

Canvas bearers with long poles, and shoulder straps, in proportion of two to every hundred men, will also be required.

2....Before a division takes the field, the principal medical officer should satisfy himself by personal inspection, that the equipment of surgeons of regiments is complete in every respect, and it would be a necessary precaution for him to see the pack horses loaded in his presence, as by that means he would ascertain that no straps, buckles, or cords were wanting.

3....When an action with the enemy seems inevitable, the surgeon of each regiment will make arrangements for the removal of the wounded of his corps from the field, and it would be desirable for him to give some instructions to the bandsmen, and others employed in that duty, how to apply a field tourniquet, to restrain dangerous hemorrhage until the assistance of the medical officer on the field can be obtained; and for this purpose a tourniquet should be given to each party of bearers. The bearers should also each of them carry a canteen full of water.

4....While the troops are advancing, the medical officers will follow with the spring wagons and bearers, and any other conveyance that is available; but when they deploy, or form for action, all, except one medical officer per regiment, will move a short distance to the rear, out of musket range, and will prepare for affording aid to the wounded, and performing such primary operations as may be deemed absolutely necessary. For this purpose the surgical panniers must be brought up, and instruments, ligatures, dressings, and cordials (brandy) got ready, and, above all things, an abundant supply of water provided, for the safe and easy conveyance of which, the leather bags, or skins, formerly recommended, would be found most convenient.

Dr. Hall takes this opportunity of cautioning medical officers against the use of chloroform, in the severe shock of serious gunshot wounds, as he thinks few will survive where it is used. But, as public opinion, founded, perhaps, on mistaken philanthropy, he knows, is against him, he can only caution medical officers, and entreat they will narrowly watch its effects, for however barbarous it may appear, the smart of the knife is a powerful stimulant, and it is much better to hear a man bawl lustily than to see him sink silently into the grave.

5. . . . One medical officer for each regiment, generally the junior assistant surgeon, should follow the troops within musket range, so as to be at hand to check any alarming hemorrhage, and to expedite the removal of the wounded off the field to the rear, and for this purpose the bearers should be placed under his orders, and the regimental spring wagon be so stationed as to be within easy reach, to convey them to where the surgeon and his assistants have established themselves. The field-assistant should carry with him, in his haversack, his pocket case of instruments, with a few ligatures ready cut, two field tourniquets, some lint, and two or three bandages; and he should be accompanied by three men, one with a knapsack, or haversack, containing one pint bottle of brandy, or some other stimulant, twenty-four bandages, half a pound of lint, three sponges, six long and six short solid splints, two old sheets cut into quarters before starting, for the purpose of rolling fractured limbs in, and so preventing them from sustaining further injury on the men's removal from the field. This is best accomplished by placing the old linen under the limb, and rolling the splint up in it from the outer edge, and rolling toward the limb on each side, and then securing the whole with two or three bands of tape. In this way Dr. Hall thinks medical officers will find they can temporarily secure fractured limbs better and much more expeditiously than in any other manner. The orderly should have in his haversack, in addition to the above articles, a piece of tape, some pins, and two or three rolls of tow. He should carry a canteen, either of wood or india-rubber, full of water, and a drinking cup. The second man should carry a canvas bearer, with shoulder straps, and, like the former, should have a canteen full of water. The third man, I think, should be armed, to protect the party against stragglers and marauders, and, like his fellows, carry a canteen full of water. The second assistant surgeon should receive the wounded from the field, see them carefully placed in the spring wagon, and then accompany the spring wagon to where the surgeon and third assistant are stationed, ready to afford them the surgical aid they may require. For

this service the second assistant surgeon should be accompanied by two men to assist in placing the men carefully in the wagon; these men should accompany the wagon, and assist in like manner in taking the wounded out. These men should likewise carry canteens full of water, and there should be a skin of water as a reserve, in the wagon, with a drinking cup.

6....The site selected by the staff-surgeon of brigade for the reception of the wounded from the field should be as sheltered as possible; and if not easily distinguished, a flag should be put up; and if any houses be near, calculated for the reception of wounded men, they should be taken possession of at once, and an abundant supply of water, and, if possible, straw provided.

7....Should the action prove decisive, tents can be pitched for the temporary accommodation of the wounded; but should the army advance, the surgeon, and one assistant, at least, should accompany their regiments, leaving one or two assistants, according to the number of wounded, to aid the divisional staff, who will pitch the reserve marquees, and make all necessary preparation for the comfort and accommodation of the wounded by having tea, broth, or essence of beef (which is readily made into broth by adding hot water), wine, and brandy, etc., ready. Should the army unfortunately meet with a reverse, all available transport must be pressed for the removal of the wounded to the rear, and they must be sent off as speedily as possible; but neither here, nor on the field of battle, should any one be carried whose hurts are so slight as to admit of his walking. Nor should commanding-officers of regiments, when wounded, be allowed to take medical officers of their own corps to the rear with them, or officers of any grade be permitted to appropriate the spring wagons for the special conveyance of themselves and their luggage; and positive orders should be given to prevent bandsmen, drummers, or pioneers, specially told off to assist the wounded, from being left in charge of officers' horses and effects.

8....Should the army have to effect a landing on an enemy's coast, with an opposing force to meet it, the men should eat a good meal before leaving the ships, and should cook whatever provisions it is necessary to serve out to them before the start. Pork is better than beef for this purpose, as it warms up more readily with any vegetable the men may find on shore. The medical officers should land with the last boats of their regiments, and should carry with them their haversacks, dressings, and canvas bearers, if the landing be opposed, so as to be able to bring the wounded at once to the boats for conveyance to the ships set apart for their reception; care should be taken that each boat employed in this service contains a supply of water and a drinking horn.

9....Should a landing be effected, and any horses be disembarked, the surgeon's pack-horse and panniers should be amongst the first.

10....As soon after an action as possible, medical officers in charge of corps will make out and transmit to the Inspector-General of hospitals, for the information of the General commanding-in-chief, returns of casualties made out agreeably to the following form:

Return of Killed and Wounded in the —— Regiment, in the Action of ——.

——	Killed.	Wounded.			Total Wounded.	Remarks.
		Dangerously.	Severely	Slightly		
Officers.						Names of officers killed and wounded to be inserted here.
Non-commissioned officers and privates.